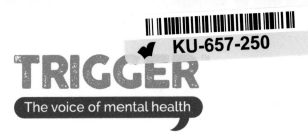

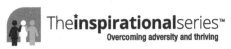
Overcoming adversity and thriving

This Too Will Pass
Anxiety in a Professional World

BY RICHARD MARTIN

We are proud to introduce The**inspirational**series™. Part of the Trigger family of innovative mental health books, The**inspirational**series™ tells the stories of the people who have battled and beaten mental health issues. For more information visit: www.triggerpublishing.com

THE AUTHOR

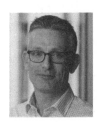
Richard Martin is a father of three mostly grown up children. He spent 20 years as a city employment lawyer, and therefore understands the pressures of professional life as well as the problems it can cause. In 2011 he suffered a series of panic attacks followed by depression and anxiety problems, which led to him being hospitalised and spending two years off work to recover.

He now works with employers in the City and elsewhere to raise awareness of mental health and wellbeing across organisations. He teaches mental health first aid, and trains managers to recognise the warning signs of developing problems, and engage in meaningful and appropriate conversations. He's on the steering committee of the Lord Mayor of London's *This is Me* campaign, which uses personal storytelling to break the stigma around mental illness. He is a qualified coach, lives in Wimbledon, has a passion for the French countryside, and spends as much time as he can outside, often on his bike.

First published in Great Britain 2018 by Trigger

Trigger is a trading style of Shaw Callaghan Ltd & Shaw Callaghan 23 USA, INC.

The Foundation Centre

Navigation House, 48 Millgate, Newark

Nottinghamshire NG24 4TS UK

www.triggerpublishing.com

Copyright © Richard Martin 2018

British Library Cataloguing in Publication Data

A CIP catalogue record for this book is available upon request
from the British Library

ISBN: 978-1-911246-41-1

This book is also available in the following e-Book and Audio formats:

MOBI: 978-1-911246-44-2
EPUB: 978-1-911246-42-8
PDF: 978-1-911246-43-5
AUDIO: 978-1-789560-48-0

Richard Martin has asserted his right under the Copyright,
Design and Patents Act 1988 to be identified as the author of this work

Cover design and typeset by Fusion Graphic Design Ltd

Printed and bound in Great Britain by Clays Ltd, Elcograf S.p.A

Paper from responsible sources

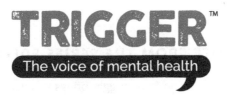

www.triggerpublishing.com

Thank you for purchasing this book.
You are making an incredible difference.

Proceeds from all Trigger books go directly to
The Shaw Mind Foundation, a global charity that focuses
entirely on mental health. To find out more about
The Shaw Mind Foundation visit,
www.shawmindfoundation.org

MISSION STATEMENT

Our goal is to make help and support available for every
single person in society, from all walks of life.
We will never stop offering hope. These are our promises.

Trigger and The Shaw Mind Foundation

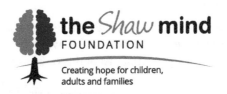

A NOTE FROM THE SERIES EDITOR

The Inspirational range from Trigger brings you genuine stories about our authors' experiences with mental health problems.

Some of the stories in our Inspirational range will move you to tears. Some will make you laugh. Some will make you feel angry, or surprised, or uplifted. Hopefully they will all change the way you see mental health problems.

These are stories we can all relate to and engage with. Stories of people experiencing mental health difficulties and finding their own ways to overcome them with dignity, humour, perseverance and spirit.

Richard Martin's moving story is about a man who "had everything", but suffered a severe depressive episode and had to rebuild his emotional wellbeing and rethink his life priorities. Richard shows us the detrimental effects of having extremely high standards, along with the dangers of over-working and ignoring signs of stress. He describes the avenues he explored in trying to understand himself and his mental health. His is an important story about challenging unhealthy approaches to mental health, and promoting self-care as a priority.

This is our Inspirational range. These are our stories. We hope you enjoy them. And most of all, we hope that they will educate and inspire you. That's what this range is all about.

Lauren Callaghan,
Co-founder and Lead Consultant Psychologist at Trigger

*To Steph, Gina, Jude and Lucy – without each of
you this book would never have been written. To Roxy for
sharing with me all your walks. And to Dr Shrew.*

Disclaimer: Some names and identifying details have been changed to protect the privacy of individuals.

Trigger encourages diversity and different viewpoints, and is dedicated to telling genuine stories of people's experiences of mental health issues. However, all views, thoughts, and opinions expressed in this book are the author's own, and are not necessarily representative of Trigger as an organisation.

INTRODUCTION

I am a father of three lovely children. I enjoy sport, good conversation, wine, food, people. I have an interest in politics and a desire to leave the world a better place than how I found it. In 2011, I was married and was enjoying a successful 20-year career as a partner in a London law firm and then, apparently without warning, I experienced a mental breakdown. This book is my story.

I hope that by telling my story I may play some small part in helping break down so much of the stigma that still surrounds mental ill health.

A primary source is a diary I kept for the first few months after my breakdown. Where I quote from that diary the text is in italics. I have sought to keep that material as close as possible to the original. The other "voices" in the book are additional narrative from the time before I was ill and after the diary stopped, my attempts to analyse or rationalise what happened, the learning I have gained and, at times, a perspective from the actual process of writing. Those voices, when they appear, should be largely clear.

Some of the material, particularly from my early childhood, is personal and raw. I have not sought to sweeten it. It is my perspective of what happened, included here because it informs what followed. It doesn't change the way I feel about the people involved now. I am not the person I was then, and neither are they.

"A breakdown isn't the beginning of mental illness, it's the publication of it. It's the volcano that has been rumbling away for years, exploding with boiling lava and destroying everything in its path. It has no choice; it was made like that, and people built houses on its slopes knowing what it was but hoping that it might not actually erupt."

Lucy Martin – 2016

CHAPTER 1

BUILDING HUMPTY'S WALL

It is said that as much as 75% of adult mental illness (excluding dementia) would be diagnosable by the age of 18, if only we looked and knew what to look for. I wonder what someone looking at me all those years ago would have seen. I did not know I was a volcano, and the eruption, when it came, was a big surprise. Looking back now, though, at all the steps and choices I have taken, there seems an inevitability to it, that I was heading inexorably to that moment in May 2011 when everything started to fall apart.

Here is a quick overview of the first 23 years of my adult life. I studied law at university. I had intended on being a barrister, the sort of lawyer that stands up in court, but I was persuaded to spend a couple of weeks on a summer placement in a solicitors' firm in the City of London. There I found interesting work and, in sharp contrast to the loneliness of my experience shadowing barristers, a sense of community and support.

And so, after law school, I joined that firm. It was, in London terms, medium-sized – probably around 200 people all told at that time. But it proudly proclaimed its difference from other firms. It punched above its weight in terms of the work it did and the clients it acted for. It had a unique training system that gave trainee solicitors (articled clerks as we were known then) far more responsibility than at other firms. Also, to attract potential recruits who might otherwise be drawn to larger firms, it had a policy of paying more than anyone else in the market. The extra money was nice, the responsibility was something I thrived on, but I think it was the sense of being different, special in some way, that really drew me in.

I worked hard and progressed well. On qualification, I joined the litigation department, which at that stage handled a huge range of different forms of dispute. I gradually started to specialise in employment work.

The firm expected you to work hard. In return, as well as the high salary, the firm made sure we could relax and have some fun. There was regularly a tab in the local pub, we had lavish summer parties, and at Christmas the younger lawyers put on a panto, an opportunity to parody the partners that ran the firm. It was a long-respected tradition, and the mark of progress in the firm, as much as being made a partner, was the moment you were first portrayed in the panto.

It was in the panto that I first met Lucy, shortly after qualification in 1995. Lucy had trained at another firm and had joined mine in the summer of that year. She worked in the corporate department. Having studied Russian and French at university, and with the Russian market just opening up to Western investment, her specialism was advising on those investment deals. She spent weeks at a time in Russia and other (ex) Soviet states. As a result, our paths had not crossed until the panto rehearsals started. I was sitting with my script, waiting for the rest of the cast to arrive for a first read through, when this confident, smiling, beautiful vision strode in. She was reading through the list of actors, working out who she knew, until she came to my initials (law firms tend to identify you by your initials).

'Who's RTM?'

'Me,' I squeaked, in awe of her already.

We got to know each other over the weeks running up to that Christmas. It took a while for us to get together, but by the new year we were an item. She was funny, intelligent, beautiful, sophisticated. There was something exotic about her Russian work. Much of her working time was spent living out of hotels in far-off places, and in London she even owned her own flat. She was a couple of years more qualified than me, which made her seem terribly grown-up, but she knew how to enjoy herself. Her fridge contained only cottage cheese and Champagne. On one occasion we had agreed to meet for lunch on one of those dead days between Christmas and New Year. She was supposed to be working that day. I had the week off. I was amazed at her audacity in staying in the pub with me all afternoon rather than going back to her desk. How brave, how cool was that? She also thought it was funny that I had a tape of Monty Python songs in my car – although perhaps she was just humouring me. And we smoked the same cigarettes – that was the clincher, clearly.

What actually was the clincher was that she was vulnerable and I seemed strong. She told me she needed a lot of looking after and I thought, *I can do that, that's what I do.* And I saw in her someone who would hold me, protect me, and love me for who I was – make me safe. We each had our unmet needs from childhood, and unconsciously thought the other could fill the hole.

She encouraged me to be brave and to explore things. I had never been outside of Europe, but she took me on holiday to Grenada – unbelievable luxury and expense. She made that seem okay, something that I was entitled to do, rather than something I did not deserve, that was for other, better people.

Things moved fast. We married in 1997 and Steph, our eldest, was born in January 1998. Lucy gave up full-time work to look after Steph – problems at work meant that she left the firm at which we met and we never really had the conversation about how we would share primary responsibility for kids. Later, she did go back to work in law firms, part-time, for a few years, but from then on, in my own head at least, I became the primary wage earner. We had been living in North London, but soon after Steph was born, moved south of the river in search of more space. It was a lonely and difficult time for Lucy with a newborn baby, a new house and neighbourhood. She didn't have any nearby friends and was left at home while I went off to work each day.

Steph, perhaps taking her cue from her parents' obvious inexperience and sharp learning curve, had been a bit shy, cautious, and uncertain as a baby. She seemed reluctant to come, arriving two weeks after her official due date, and just before she was going to be induced. She looked like us too, with her thick brown hair and olive skin, as if she had taken on Lucy's love of the sun.

When Gina arrived in August 2000, she could not have been more different. Born two weeks early, she burst upon the world with an exuberance of ginger hair and smiles. Her skin was porcelain white and her eyes stayed blue. We had had vague conversations about how many kids we might want to have; at least three seemed to be the understanding. Gina was such an easy baby. She slept at every opportunity and seemed to smile with such delight. And before we had finished thinking about whether and when we might try for a third, we were pregnant with Jude.

Jude was due in April 2002. By this stage my career was flying, and I was being considered for promotion to partnership in the spring of that year. I felt the pressure to get the promotion and was working long hours to achieve it. At the time I would have said it was about providing for my growing family but there were myriad other motivations at play. Steph was the ripe old age of four, Gina 18 months. We had our hands full.

Then, early in that year, Lucy got a chest infection. Increasingly pregnant, tired, and weak with the chest infection, she spent a lot of time in bed. The infection worsened and developed into pleurisy, pneumonia and, finally, blood clots on her lungs.

Diagnoses were missed, and the problems were exacerbated by the fact that when she was hospitalised, as happened on a regular basis, she would be admitted to a maternity ward where the focus was on the baby, who was fine, rather than Lucy, who was not.

My memories of those months are of juggling longs hours at work with a home life which was a mix of hospital, sick bed, friends picking up children and general angst about Lucy's state of health.

In the end, Jude was safely delivered in April, but Lucy was still very ill. With him out, the doctors could give her the medication she needed for the blood clots. She slowly recovered her strength. By the summer, she was getting back on her feet. At an outpatient appointment, a doctor who had been involved in her care before the birth happened to pass by us, smiled and said, 'So you made it then!' We had known she was seriously ill, but I don't think I had registered it was quite as touch-and-go as that.

Later that summer, my promotion long since granted, I was leaving the office one evening. There had been a drinks reception at which I had had to make an appearance, but I left as early as I could. I needed to get some money out of an ATM, but I could not make it work. I tried a few times but got into an increasing frenzy until I found myself sitting on the pavement crying, unable to keep myself together. I managed to call one of my colleagues and asked her to help get me home, which she did. I think the pressure of the previous months had just built and built. Once I knew that Lucy was through the worst, it was as if I could finally let go of the strain and breathe, and I collapsed in a bit of a heap.

I took a couple of weeks off work. The doctor prescribed some mild anti-depressant medication and suggested some therapy, both of which I stuck at for a few months until the symptoms passed. Putting it all down to the combination of pressure from everything going on at the time, I never really thought about it again.

That was a mistake.

As the years passed we did more and more. We extended our first house and then bought a bigger one, which we also extended. We had big parties. Lucy would organise a busy social life. She encouraged the children in music and art, so the house was filled with instruments and paintings and noise and people. And all the while, I was taking on more and more roles and responsibilities.

A partner in a city law firm gets paid a load of money which funds a comfortable lifestyle, but you sure have to work hard for it. The hours are long and pressured. There are never-ending demands from clients and your team. You are constantly running at a hundred miles an hour, spinning multiple plates as you go.

I remember one Monday morning leaving to go to work and Gina was at the top of the stairs as I turned to say goodbye. 'Goodbye Daddy, see you on Saturday.' I wasn't travelling anywhere, I just never managed to get home in time to see her before she went to bed. So, when I was home I tried to do as much as I could with them all, as well as in the house and garden.

At the same time, I was also saying yes to anyone who asked for my help or my time. As an employment lawyer, you are always in demand for informal advice from friends. But when some locals decided to set up a residents' association, I agreed to chair it. When a friend wanted a new chair for a local civic forum, flattered by the request, I agreed. When the kids' school asked me to join the governing body, I agreed. When the church wanted help, I said yes. When it came to Christmas and our friend was organising a lunch for a hundred or more people who would otherwise be on their own on Christmas Day, we agreed to help out. When you are the professional lawyer in the wider family, it is you that is asked to look at wills, or take on powers of attorney, or look at this or that agreement. And you do it because it is expected of you, because you have been asked, because it is the right thing to do.

It was as if I was constantly trying to prove myself worthy, that, with each new badge and role, I was seeking some kind of recognition of worth, of value. Somehow there was no sense of me, but merely what I did. If I had ever had any sense of me, of who I was, I was losing it in this frantic frenzy of activity.

And of course, it all takes its toll in terms of time. My job was demanding enough but I was heaping all this other stuff on too, further reducing what was left for Lucy, the family, or me.

Lucy describes me in the years leading up to 2011 as like an increasingly stretched elastic band. She was getting more and more unhappy with the ways things were, while my solution was to plough on and hope it would be alright in the end. After all, I was doing the right thing, wasn't I, working hard and all that? I moved to a different law firm and got involved in management of the firm which brought more responsibility, more demands, and another badge. Increasingly I could not cope with Lucy's unhappiness. When she would try to tell me how bad things were, I struggled to hear or listen lest the elastic band snapped.

At work, clients and colleagues would bring me problems and I would help solve them. That was my job, they were grateful, and I got a pat on the back. I could not solve the problems at home, so I sought to shut them out. There were times when it was a relief to leave for work in the morning and I would fear phoning Lucy from work lest her growing unhappiness with me disrupt the comparative calm of the office. I felt that in telling me of her unhappiness, Lucy was expecting me to sort it out – and perhaps she was to an extent – making it my responsibility, my fault. All I could think was that I was doing all I could. What more could she or anyone expect from me? I just had to get my head down and carry on.

I remember two regular dreams from that period. In one, someone (perhaps me) was diving from a high board. The diver would go into a series of somersaults through the air as he fell towards the water, but he could not get out of the spin, could not straighten out for entry into the pool. He just kept on spinning, the water getting ever closer, but never quite reaching the splash point. In the other dream, there was an ice skater pirouetting. The spin would get faster and faster and, like the diver, the skater just could not stop the spin. I did not reflect on the dreams at the time, but looking back, they were clearly reflecting the unsustainably frantic nature of my life – I was spinning out of control.

No one on the outside saw any of this apart from Lucy. And I was not listening to what she was saying. To the outside world I appeared to have a charmed existence. A beautiful wife, three perfect children, a great job, good prospects. Earlier that year we had bought a holiday cottage in the French countryside. And I was popular at work, I think. I was the one that seemed able to take on anything and cope, excel even. I had made it.

Sometimes, however, the brighter the light, the deeper the shadow.

CHAPTER 2

BUT, RICHARD, WHAT DO YOU WANT?

In early 2011, my firm suggested that in preparation for my next promotion, it might benefit me to see an executive coach. *Why not?* I thought, having no real idea what coaching entailed but feeling secretly honoured that this investment was being made in me. Six sessions were planned, two hours each, over the course of a few months. The coach would come to our office and we would sit and talk. It felt pretty strange, at the time, to be having deeply personal conversations in the same meeting rooms where I usually saw clients or colleagues.

Early on, I did a psychometric test. When the coach presented the results to me, he began by asking me whether I ever felt different to the people around me in the law firm, whether there were times when I thought they did not understand me, or I did not understand them. 'Of course,' I replied. 'That's normal isn't it?'

Apparently it isn't. Apparently, most people don't think like that for much of the time. Hmm ...

He showed me a graph to illustrate the point. He drew a curve to show the average, normal personality traits of a lawyer, and then he superimposed my curve on the top. They were almost polar opposites.

'Now these are only based on norms,' he said, 'and I am not saying for a moment that you aren't a good lawyer, but this may go some way to explain why you have that sense of difference, of not quite belonging. You are just very different to many of the people around you.'

Later he said he'd got a clear understanding of what the firm wanted of me, why it saw the potential it did in me, and why he had been asked to work with me. 'But what I want to know, Richard, is what do you want?'

And I just did not understand the question.

I had a wife and family to support, a mortgage, school fees, a department to run, and a mapped-out career path to follow. 'What do you mean, what do I want?' And as he looked kindly into my eyes and repeated the question, I began to realise for the first time in many, many years that I, Richard, had a choice. I could ask myself what I wanted and, to an extent at least, it was reasonable to try to achieve that.

As I write that, I am overcome with emotion. Apparently, the part of our brain that deals with emotion cannot support language – it works in images rather than words. This book, this collection of words, is all about feelings and emotion. There is, therefore, a lot of translation to be done between me recalling emotions and you understanding them. First, I have to translate images in my head into language. You will then take my words and form your own interpretation of what I have said. Finally, you will translate those words into images that will make sense to your brain.

As a result, I have little sense of whether the enormity of what I felt at the time, and still feel now, is remotely conveyed by the words I have used. A metaphor might help, one which I have thought about a lot over recent years. Imagine building a big house. You start with the foundations and then build on top of that, never giving another thought to those foundations. They are just taken for granted as you build and change and develop and extend over the years, until you end up with a massive structure sitting on those foundations. And then one day you realise the foundation is fatally flawed. The basis upon which everything else has been built, the assumption that it was all a matter of doing your duty (and that what you wanted or felt did not matter at all) is false.

It didn't take long for the cracks to start appearing. I think that conversation was in my fifth session with the coach and I never made it to the sixth. I went away with the family for the May half-term holiday to France and I never went back to work again.

I should say that I am a huge supporter of coaching. I just had no idea what was going to come of it and was unprepared as a result. It started me on a journey that I needed to take somehow, to a destination that is still unclear to me. Living with that degree of uncertainty is one of the biggest challenges I am still trying to learn to deal with.

CHAPTER 3

FUNNY TURNS
IN THE CHARENTE

For as long as I can remember, I have had intermittent "funny turns". They are hard to describe. I get thoughts coming into my head – places, people, and voices. In the moment, they seem so very familiar to me that it feels like they must have happened somehow, somewhere, some time, but I just cannot put my finger on how, where, or when. Afterwards it is hard to remember any real detail other than the very clear sense that the images are fantastical. The familiarity then becomes hard to explain – are they a dream I am remembering, or are they simply the same voices and images from previous episodes that become more familiar each time? Or am I recalling elements of some traumatic event that I have otherwise blocked from memory?

The images and thoughts are welcoming, enticing, inviting. They want me to give in to them and let them take over my head – it is a struggle to resist the lure of going with them, if only to try to find out what they are and why they are familiar. Normally, when I get an episode of this, it happens a few more times over a day or two. The first episode I can just about push back and resist if I am in a place where I cannot give in – I know what is coming so it is dangerous if I am driving, or in a meeting or something.

The thoughts will come back though and, when they do, and I let them in, they overwhelm my head and I can think of nothing else. And then I come over all faint as if the blood has been sucked out of me, or my blood pressure has dropped dramatically at least, and I have to sit or hold on to something. Once I am at that point, the sensation lasts for a few minutes. I do not lose consciousness and I do not lose connection with the world – I can talk to people around me. After a minute or two I am okay again, but I know that I am in a run of such episodes and the thoughts will return before too long.

As you can imagine, it's quite a scary experience. I had always associated them with tiredness because when I mentioned them to my mum once, that's what she said. I generally found that if I lay down and got some sleep, or got an early night, the funny turns would stop. Later, when I mentioned them to my psychiatrist, he was very interested in them, and I ended up having them investigated by a neurologist who suggested they might be a form of mild partial seizure of some kind, but not quite on the epileptic spectrum.

My own view now is that it wasn't tiredness, but rather anxiety. It's clear that the two can often go hand-in-hand and feed off each other. Poor sleep can contribute to anxiety and anxiety can cause poor sleep. Anxiety is a fear reaction, your body responding to a perceived threat which we are pre-programmed to respond to in a physical way – classically flight or fight (although freeze and fold are additional possible reactions). If you are faced with a tiger that's about to attack, it's not a great idea to fall asleep! My understanding now is that those "funny turns" were in fact moments where my anxiety was overwhelming me, small scale panic attacks in effect.

We were spending a week's holiday in May 2011 at our house in the Charente countryside. Previously, we had always taken an overnight ferry from Portsmouth to Caen, leaving a five-

or six-hour drive the following morning. This time, however, we had decided to give the Channel tunnel a try. The Channel crossing would be much shorter, although it meant the drive the other side would be more like seven hours.

Once we arrived, I started getting my funny turns. This time, however, rather than being many hours apart as was the norm, they were happening every hour, or even more regularly, and no amount of sleep would make them go away.

On one occasion we were at a brocante, basically an upmarket French version of our car boot sales. They close the town centre off to traffic and, for a small fee, you can book a stall and sell whatever you like. Some people make a living out of selling stuff there. Most seem to regard it either as a social occasion, or as an alternative to the local dump. In fact, it often seems like someone has removed the entire contents of the dump and distributed it to the stall holders with a challenge to see what they can make of it. The organisers keep the stall holders supplied with a steady flow of local brew, Pineau, and it's basically a social occasion with the odd bit of negotiating along the way. In my imagination, at the end of the day they bring the skips back and all the junk gets put back in and returned to the dump until the next time.

The five of us were wandering around when I had one of my turns, and ended up sitting on the ground, at which point one of the kindly stall holders let me lie down in the back of his van and found me a glass of water. As you will have gathered, it's hard enough to try to explain these episodes in English – doing so in French was well-nigh impossible. I suspect he assumed I had had a bit too much Pineau.

Eventually, about halfway through the week, the funny turns stopped. The rest of the week passed fairly uneventfully. I was pretty busy doing work around the land, mowing grass, chopping trees, clearing overgrown areas – the sort of physical activity I enjoy and get satisfaction from. As is my tendency, I did rather more work than was probably necessary or helpful.

On the final Saturday, for example, I was clearing up some garden waste and taking it to the compost heap near the (empty) stable. The approach to the stable was overgrown with brambles and so I thought I would clear a path through the brambles to the stable.

What began as a little bit of work that might have taken a few minutes turned in to several hours, as the area I decided to clear became ever larger, me losing all sense of proportion. There is a lot of land around the house – low grade agricultural land in the middle of nowhere is cheap in France. Clearing a few square metres of brambles at one side of one field was really not going to make a difference to anyone. It was the last day of the break and there really might have been better things to spend my time on (playing with the kids, maybe) than hacking away at brambles, exhausting work as it was. There was a small amount of satisfaction to be had, but nothing like the pain involved to achieve it.

Although I can recall elements of that trip, there is much that I cannot remember at all ... When we had bought the house, it had a very old pool and there are photos of us all working hard to empty it, clean it out and refill it, and then of us using it. I am in those photos, but I have no recollection of any of that. I have stared at the photos repeatedly, trying to stir up the memories that must be there somewhere – we were smiling, they were happy times – but I just cannot make any connection between the man who looks like me in the photos, and what I remember.

Une Pomme Anglaise

We drove back on the Sunday.

We were running late and the sat nav had given us duff directions to go round the périphérique instead of avoiding Paris like the plague, but we were not too stressed about it. I had been doing all the driving but had had two stops and was quite happy. Around 2.30pm or so, an hour after the last stop,

I started feeling a little "not right" – slightly nauseous, slightly tired, enough to make me think I would ask Lucy to take over driving when we were next able to stop, but it was not an emergency.

We came towards a péage gate and suddenly I felt very nauseous, very panicky, and desperate to get out of the car. I got out where we were and told Lucy to take over driving. I tried to get into the passenger seat and got as far as sitting and closing the door, but I was in a blind panic and could not stay there. My heart was beating hard and fast. I got out and walked towards the gate up the line of traffic, then skipped across endless lanes towards what looked like the office. I felt very scared, very alone, not knowing what to do or what was happening. I was stopped by a lady attendant from crossing the automated télépéage lanes where vehicles do not stop and she sat me down in the shade of the gate cover between the lanes of traffic. They then closed the télépéage lanes and I walked over to the office.

They gave me water, I think, and at some stage Lucy joined me but I am not sure when. They called the pompiers (the firemen seem to double up as paramedics) and a van and two other vehicles soon arrived. They were quite comical – deciding after a while to take my pulse and then finding someone with a watch, a pen, a scrap of paper. They asked me had I eaten something odd. I was with it enough to joke with them that I had eaten an English apple which must have been the cause. "Ah oui, monsieur, bien sur c'est la pomme Anglaise".

They advised I go to hospital which I did in the back of the van. They did ECG tests three times, blood tests and a chest x-ray and found nothing untoward. My heart had calmed and I was feeling better. We left after around two and a half hours.

What I remember finding comical was how the doctor said that when I got back to England I should go and see my cardiologist – my cardiologist you understand, not just any cardiologist, because we all have our own one of them, don't we? But maybe you do in France. They always strike me as a kinder race – kinder to themselves as well as others, so it may be no coincidence that they take good care of their hearts.

I now know that what I had experienced was a panic attack. From the outside it can look very like a heart attack which is obviously more immediately dangerous, so the form is to assume that's what it is and assess for heart problems. Thankfully that was not the problem. There was no suggestion, as far as I was aware, of any other likely cause of the symptoms.

The journey home from there was a nightmare. We had missed our scheduled train and there was a storm over France which made the driving horrible. Lucy had found out that the next available train was at 10.30pm and the one after that not until 1.30am. Steph had exams in the morning. She was already going to struggle for a good night's sleep, but a 1.30am train would have been a disaster. Lucy did all the driving from that point and we did make the 10.30 train, just. There were storms, and it was dark, on the English side and we finally got home and into bed around 1.00am.

That detail is all from notes in my diary. I don't remember much of it (and I have no recollection of how the exam went).

CHAPTER 4

WHAT'S HAPPENING TO ME?

I phoned my GP in the morning. It was the start of a long and very helpful relationship with Dr Murray. There must also have been some toing and froing involved to allow me actually to speak to him on the phone – it's not like we had a direct line – and there's no way I would have managed that, so I am guessing Lucy sorted it all.

Dr Murray quickly discounted any issue with my heart and suggested that anxiety may be the cause. He suggested we see how things settled over the following days and recommended I look at a local counselling service.

The next days were awful.

Everything seemed to be lived through a haze of treacle. Seeing, hearing, smelling, thinking, walking, feeling, everything enveloped in a haze of treacle and a massive effort as a result. My short-term memory has gone, and I am waking at 4.00am each day and am exhausted. Lucy tells me what to do, she feeds me, tells me what is happening, tells me names and places. She determines what happens where and when, but with a kindness and gentleness. She has taken charge and I am dependent on her in a way I never imagined. I dare not go out. When people come to the door I cower in the shadows behind Lucy. I feel like a non-sentient beast. Too big and too lumbering for what little purpose it might have, having to be led by the nose, grunting.

I have blown a fuse. My brain and body are not functioning properly – perhaps operating on emergency power only – keeping me alive but nothing more.

I am scared. I do not understand what is happening. I have never felt this way before. I assume I have had a breakdown of some sort. The GP did not rule out something viral and so I keep that as a possibility for a while, but I know it's not likely.

I sit and read if I can, but cannot manage more than a few pages at once. Lucy buys me a jigsaw of London – 1,000 pieces – which I become obsessed over and finish in a few days.

The strange thing is that I do manage to do some work. I field emails, redirecting work. I have calls with an assistant on the latest events on cases. I go through draft witness statements and discuss changes with another assistant, and I review a draft settlement agreement and am able to discuss it with the client. These are all single tasks which I can do in bursts, in my own time.

I do a lot of crying. The Thursday of the first week was particularly bad. I had cried a bit during the day, for no apparent reason most of the time. Then I had supper with the kids and at about half- seven I just started crying and could not stop and Gina put me tenderly to bed.

That scared the kids so I talked to them the following day to try to reassure them, but I do not know if I was successful. I have started using the home computer and Lucy's email address, so I end up catching glimpses of emails she is sending to friends talking about worries that she does not let on to me – when will I get better, if I don't go back to my old job can we afford the mortgage, school fees etc.

Dr Murray referred me to a consultant psychiatrist at the Priory. The consultant had no appointments until mid-July and there was some confusion between me and Dr Murray trying to source someone else. I must have made some of these calls myself; I remember clearly how even a simple phone call needed a ten-minute build-up to overcome the attendant anxiety, then left me panicking throughout, and for a good period afterwards.

I also saw a homeopath on the Wednesday, I think, who gave me various potions, largely to deal with fatigue, feeling overwhelmed, and the liver. I did start to improve but who knows what would have happened anyway.

I saw a reiki healer on the Friday which knocked me out – amazing feelings of calmness and peace and her hands felt hot on my back.

I remember Lucy sorting out these appointments and taking me there. I would have to ask her again and again where we were going, why, and who we were going to see. I remember not being able to speak above a whisper and needing her by my side the whole time, leading me gently, being my support, and terrified if she left me alone with someone else.

The frustration with not getting a consultant through the GP, and also the need to update work, meant I gave them the full story of what had happened so far. HR immediately sprang into effective action – it is amazing what strings they can pull and resources they can mobilise when needed. So, they sorted an occupational health appointment for Thursday next week and, on the basis that I am likely to need it, a consultant psychiatrist at the Priory for the Friday. So that is reassuring and makes me feel like someone else is helping and things are likely to start happening – that there is the beginning of a plan.

That first week was like a blur – everything out of focus, nothing functioning, fatigue, overwhelmed, childlike, scared, crying, not sleeping at night, totally dependent on Lucy. Watching the world go on around me while playing no part in it.

Dad came for a visit some time in this week. I cannot imagine what he was thinking or whether he had any understanding of what was happening to me. Of the three of us boys, I had been the one who had seemed to fulfil his ambitions – top university, success in a profession, the wealth that comes with it. Then this.

What had happened? If I had not seen it coming, he certainly would not have seen any warning signs. There was a history of mental illness in his family, and from a time when sufferers were treated rather less kindly than they are today. Perhaps memories of that were being stirred up in him, I don't know. In any event, he was calm, gentle, and tender. He listened and that was enough.

The Saturday of that week, still the first week after the panic attack, was the local school family day. The school is literally across the road from where we lived. As well as being a parent to three kids who had been (or were going) through the school, I had also been a governor for many years, so I knew a lot of people there. It ought to have been a safe place and the family day is a celebration, a time to relax and have fun.

I am dreading it. I cannot imagine how I will be able to talk to anyone. I am scared, I don't know what to say, I don't know what people know about what has happened. It's as if people will see me but I won't be there. There is nothing inside me but treacle. But Lucy encourages me to go over for a bit, to see what I can manage.

Around 12 I wander over for an hour and stay close to Lucy or one of the kids. I cannot risk being on my own. I manage about an hour then come back home and watch the TV – whatever sport was on, I think. It's exhausting being out in the world and terrified by it. Later we went round to some friends for an impromptu drink. My plan had not been to stay long – that was a precondition of me agreeing that I could manage it in the first place – but I end up staying until after 9pm. It's somewhere safe and it is reassuring to be seeing people and feeling part of the world.

At some stage that day I drove the car for the first time – just five minutes up the road to fetch a friend's kid from a party. Then something happened which makes so much difference. It's a truism about mental health that we don't talk about it. We don't learn about it at school and, historically, mental illness was a subject of shame. So when it happens to you, first of all you have no idea what is going on. Secondly, you assume that, because no one else you know has ever spoken to you about this kind of stuff, you are the only one. How wrong can you be? I don't know whether he had been tipped off by Lucy, or whether I told him what was happening, or he recognised it himself, but the father from whom I was collecting the kid told me all sorts of stories from his childhood and the various episodes of mental problems he has had through his life.

This happens to other people, people who seem better, able to manage life again. There are people who have a sense of what I am experiencing, they understand and can talk about it. It is such a relief.

Week 2

Over the next week, sleep got a little better – waking at five rather than four most mornings. I am crying less often perhaps, but crying is still very much there. I have a bit more energy and am feeling a little more able to do things for myself and cope on my own. Lucy goes out a couple of evenings and it's okay. Monday and Tuesday, I walk the dogs, Monday on my own and Tuesday with Lucy. Both times it's tiring and stressful.

I am drinking every night – it gets to 7pm and I need a drink. I drink a bit of coffee – I had avoided it all last week. I am smoking too much but there's so little to do to take your mind off things. I try to avoid thinking / talking about the future other than in very immediate terms.

I am still doing work from home – a couple of hours a day maybe at most.

I can't do more than one thing a day – some work, a walk, the doctor, whatever. Just one thing.

Being ill, mentally ill, can be really tiring. You have to accept that and go with it. I tried to remain as active as I could, however limited that was, to maintain some degree of purpose and connection with the world. At the same time you have to be kind to, and listen to, yourself. If you broke your leg, you would expect to have to spend a lot of time doing nothing. It's the same thing. There is also the whole sleep cycle thing. You are exhausted from the illness and all you want to do is sleep, but the one thing your body won't do is let you have it.

Another thing that took some getting used to was thinking about the future. We can all get very used to thinking long-term, planning this and that. When your world has fallen apart, you are desperate to want to work out how to rebuild it, to know when you will be better, to think about how you return to work, to have some certainty. Gradually you realise that you have to let that all go, at least for a while. Sometimes just being alive the next day, or out of bed, is enough of a long-term plan, and quite an achievement too.

It's also reassuring to notice that even though you have not done all the things you normally do, all the busy little things you contribute to the world, the sun has still come up and gone down, the world has turned, the tides have done their thing, everyone around you has eaten and the roof is still where it should be atop the house. Some of those things might have happened because someone else shouldered the burden. Let them. Thank them and remember what they did. But let them do it because there will be times when you just can't.

Inevitably, there are some things you do have to do, but you need to give yourself more time and care in doing them. On the Thursday of that second week I had to go to Central London to attend the appointment with occupational health. I was in a right old state worrying about how I was going to get there. I had been there before for various health check-ups in the past, but I lacked any confidence in being able to remember the way and had to keep focused on how I would manage it. This became a constant thing for me with any journey, particularly involving public transport.

I carefully planned my route – it wasn't complicated. I just had to get a train to Waterloo then get on the Waterloo and City line to Bank – but I needed a piece of paper to remind me that was what I had to do, and how to walk from Bank to the surgery.

I was also terrified about being on the train. I am not sure what was scary about it – the people, I guess – but I borrowed an iPod so that I could listen to music and shut the world out. Even now, public transport is a problem for me quite often and so I make sure I have a book to engross myself in if I need to shut the world away.

Lucy drove me to the station – I did not feel up to the 10-minute walk and she was probably worried about whether I would make it. The train and Tube journeys were shaky but manageable with my music. The walk from Bank was really hard, however. This was where I worked, my manor, but now it terrified me. All these buildings I used to walk into without a thought, all these people in suits; I used to be part of that, but now it seemed another world to me, and not a friendly one. All very surreal and out of kilter. I had this immense feeling of not belonging, of being an alien, and I was terrified.

I arrived half an hour early for the appointment, so I had to sit and wait. I was worried about seeing someone from my work there so tried to hide myself in a corner. The doctor I saw was very kind, understanding, and pragmatic. I cried a lot. She instructed me to stop all work. She made it feel okay and normal. She made a point of looking me in the eye – and forcing me to look her in the eye – to say I will get better. She told me not to think about the medium-term and confirmed that, in her view, I had experienced an anxiety episode and that I should see the psychiatrist the next day.

I was exhausted afterwards, but that evening I signed off from work – I gave details of all my files to the other partners in the team and confirmed that I was doing nothing more. I also looked at the last two witness statements for one of my assistants and talked to her about them before telling her that was it – she was on her own now and if she needed more support she would need to talk to one of the other partners.

Although I had not been doing much work, or been able to do much work, I had tried to do the bits I felt most responsible for and this meant a constant worry in my head about needing to keep on top of it all. Saying to the world of work that I was downing tools completely was a blessed relief. One day your head is filled with all the work issues that keep you occupied and then the next day none of it matters. Not just for the week(s) you go on holiday, but for as long as it takes – just give it all up. I didn't have to care any more and I didn't care. Of course, it had taken a firm instruction from a medic to make me do that, to give me the permission to do what ought to have been blindingly apparent was the right thing to do, but nonetheless I got there in the end.

The appointment with the psychiatrist involved a similar amount of angst and planning over the longer journey to the Priory in Southgate, North London.

The psychiatrist was middle aged, a little older than me, I guess, slightly balding, a little dishevelled. There was a reassuring sense that he knew what human misery is like. He was respectful of it, and of me. He was curious, wondering. He was also empathetic and at the same time confident – he did not skirt around my condition but strode briskly towards it.

He took details of my case history – I was getting used to this by now. He was particularly interested in my funny turns – 'Something does not stack up, I am not happy, it does not fit together,' he tells me. I am thinking, What? Is this all a sham, have I been making this all up and he has seen through me? *but what he meant was that he wanted to get to the bottom of the funny turns. 'They might be mild epilepsy and it would be foolish not to try to understand and get to the bottom of that before moving forward with therapy, not least because any therapy or medication might exacerbate epilepsy.' As a result, he referred me to a neurologist for some tests. I get home with an enthusiasm born of there being a plan, that something is happening, and I can play my part in it.*

I am reading a book on depression [Depressive Illness – The Curse of the Strong, referred to in more detail later]. *It is very helpful and reassuring – it talks about depression as a physical disease caused by chemical imbalance and that the honest, morally robust, hard workers are most likely to get stress-induced depression because they do not stop or give in – they take more and more of what they are asked to do, carry on, carry on until one day their body snaps – a fuse is blown. The book has a suggested time plan for the week, with time set aside for different tasks and with clear time for relaxation and hobbies – what has happened to mine? I have just worked and worked and done school governors and other stuff and never stopped, leaving me, my wife, and my family to suffer – where in the pecking order did they come? Why was work more important than them? Who has set all the rules by which I am trying to live? Who am I trying to impress? What do I want – me, really me, what do I want? On the one hand, these thoughts are all there and pressing on me while at the same time I am told by the doctors not to think about the bigger picture. The psychiatrist told me very politely that I was in no state to be thinking about longer-term things like that. He is also very clear he does not want me working.*

It is surprisingly easy and quite liberating to hand over work and not to have anything more to do with it. I no longer have any conflict in my day as to what I should be doing – do nothing. It does make the thought of a return to work more difficult because I am that much further away from it.

I begin to worry about getting better – that if I do, that might mean I have to go back to work which I cannot cope with, but that is circular isn't it? If I am better, then I will be able to cope. It's too confusing in my head.

Short-term memory is a problem. I have to write lists and tick things off as quickly as possible lest I forget tasks. I have bits of paper all over the place with things written on them.

One of the things I recall strongly from the many meetings with the psychiatrist over the first year or so was that, although he recognised I was broken, and allowed me to be broken, to cry, to not know the answers, he always gave the sense of knowing that I had not always been like this. This was just the illness.

Although I never knew him before I was ill, it felt like he could see through the illness to a well me. He would make a point of telling me that this will get better, that he has seen this before and it will improve. He would never say when or by how much, but, always, that it would improve.

One of the themes from those early days is having little idea what was happening to me, but then sometimes finding someone who had had similar experiences and the relief of knowing I was not alone. By now I know the statistics and appreciate just how common problems are. I can get on a bus and estimate how many of my fellow passengers are likely to be suffering from a serious mental health condition right now.

Perhaps most importantly, I can look people in the eye sometimes and see something in them that tells me that yes, you too have known what it is to be broken, to not function at all. You too have looked over the cliff, real or imagined, and seen the void and wanted to embrace it because it's all there is. You too have looked into the mirror of your mind and seen only a jumbled mass of spaghetti, and not recognised yourself, and feared that you had gone forever. It is a privilege when you meet someone like that, and a comfort. Conversations move quickly beyond the weather ...

I cannot emphasise enough just how important talking about how we are can be. If you are suffering from problems, no matter how serious they may be, talking to people helps. It helps you to understand things for yourself when you try to articulate them for others, forcing you to recognise what is really happening for you and sometimes bringing some perspective to bear. Connection with people is a vital component of looking after your wellbeing. Knowing that you have the permission to talk to people about how you are is an immense relief. While it's great if the person you are talking to has some understanding of mental health problems, it does not matter if they don't. All they need to do, all any of us need to do, is to listen, and to listen compassionately.

How many conversations do we have every day that go something along the lines of:

'Hi, how are you?'

'Fine. You?'

'All good thanks. Anyway ...' and you then move on to what you really wanted to talk about or you carry on with whatever you were doing.

When someone asks how we are, we feel obliged to gloss over it or tell them what we assume they want to hear. How would it be if, even just once each day, we took the time to answer the question properly? Maybe they don't actually want to know, and if you make a point of actually telling them, they might stop asking. Or perhaps they'll realise it's a good thing to have asked and obtain a sense of connection with you.

One time a family friend asked me how I was, and I was giving the normal answer when she looked at me and said, 'But you're not really fine, are you?' When I realised the permission I had to tell her the truth it was such a relief. She didn't provide any answers, she didn't make things better, she had no magic wand, but that didn't matter. The fact that she cared enough to want to know and told me with her eyes and her tenderness that it was okay to be broken and to tell her that, was more than enough.

One of the strong memories of the first several months, and in particular the first weeks, is the fear of the phone ringing. If I had to make a phone call myself then I would spend ages gearing myself up to do it, and finding reasons to postpone it, in order to feel that I could carry the conversation off, remember what I wanted to say, what I wanted to get out of the conversation, and not break down in tears. When the phone rang, the noise of the ringing, like any sudden noise, would cause me to jump out of whatever chair I was slumped in and create huge agitation. But worse was the fear that someone would be wanting to talk to me. It did not matter whether it was a friend, family, work, the doctor's surgery, whoever. I could not face a conversation without the necessary preparation.

It is a common problem for those who know people with mental health problems – you want to talk to them, see how they are, be kind and supportive, but they are terrified of talking to you. There is nothing you can do but keep trying, leave positive messages and hope they will ring you back. Sometimes agreeing a time to speak is good so that the person can get ready for the call and knows who it will be when the phone rings – and of course mobiles are good with their call identification, so you can at least know who it is before you take the call.

It is still a problem for me. I rarely answer calls from numbers I do not recognise, preferring to let the person leave a message so I can call them back once I know who they are.

CHAPTER 5

THE PERILS OF SUPERMARKETS

Whenever I had a busy day, the next was sure to be really hard – feeling the exhaustion and with anxiety levels turned up many degrees. On Monday 20th June I had been very brave and had gone to watch the end of a cricket match. Here's Tuesday:

Today is a treacle day. I knew last night it was going to be. I tried to do too much yesterday and yesterday evening I was feeling just a little vulnerable and quite tired, so I knew today was going to be hard.

I know that I need to give in to the day and do very little. Do not try to be over ambitious – I do not need to achieve anything today other than get through the day with as little damage to my surroundings as possible. Not crying would be good, but probably unrealistic.

I shave, because most mornings I try either to shower or shave – doing both is normally beyond me, but doing one or the other stops me having another reason to feel cut off and miserable. Somehow it helps me feel connected with what everyone else is doing and what I normally do.

Today is a day for doing not very much at all. I ask Lucy if there is anything she needs me to do and she mentions Daddy's mending box in the playroom. I have a slight panic because I did not know there was a Daddy's mending box and so the contents may go back some time if the other members of the family have been used to popping all their broken things in there for more than a few weeks. As it turns out, it is nicely manageable – a series of small tasks that can be completed one at a time and each takes little time and little brain power or physical exertion – just right for a day like today. To create a kind of check list and to create a sense of achievement, I lay them out in a row and then when completed move them to a different row. I take the easy ones first:

1. A pirate "Keep Out" sign made out of clay and painted by Jude that belongs on his bedroom door but which fell off some time ago and broke in two. It is a job for superglue. It is a relief to find it without too much effort. I manage to make the fix without sticking the sign to the table or my fingers and proudly move it to the finished pile;

2. A football which needs pumping up – this could be a disaster if the things I need are not where they should be, but they are, and the ball is soon a familiar shape – things are going well;

3. A light that needs a new bulb – I go up to the office in the loft and I remember the two bulbs in the bathroom that need replacing and do them on the way back. These are not complicated tasks but ones that could easily go inconsolably wrong in my present state. Even when the old bulb breaks in my hand as I try to unscrew it, I manage to keep myself together;

4. Some other lights need new batteries and I feel good about myself that I bought some of that very size just at the weekend, so we have them AND I know where they are;

5. A couple of handheld electronic games need watch batteries – that is beyond my limited battery stock. I think about whether I could go to a shop today to buy them – on the plus side it would be a great achievement and would show the game owners that I have done something today. On the downside I cannot imagine being able to cope with the combination of writing down what I need, going to the shop, parking either the car or my bike, going

into the shop, working out (or even worse having to ask for) what I need, paying for it and then getting home again. A task that normally is one job – go and buy the batteries we need – becomes an almost endless series of mini tasks each of which feels like a mountain today. No, that will be a job for another day and I am forced to concede that I will not finish my box of Daddy mending things today, and it will sit half-finished, reminding me for several days until I get to the battery shop. But it will have to fight for space in the increasingly crowded half-done category.

The things that defeat me completely are a lava lamp that offers only one way in via some screws on the bottom, over which is stuck a label saying do not open, and a wind-up clock made from a kit a while back. It worked then but I think the spring mechanism is gone and I ask Lucy's permission to bin them both which she gladly gives me. Of course, I do not get around to actually binning them and so later when I sit down to write this, I realise Lucy has done so as part of clearing the table for her teaching.

I also manage to cut the edges of the lawn – Lucy mowed it yesterday and in fact the edges were not done the last time it was cut either. It's a job that is 10 minutes at normal times – round the edge of the lawn, round the shed and decking, the washing line and the trampoline. Today I do it in about five instalments, each interspersed with a sit down.

I also keep stopping because there is a courier coming from work to take back a client file. This trivial interaction with the office and the wider world takes on ridiculous proportions. I worry about not hearing the door and the courier going back empty handed, me having wasted his time and failed in the pretty simple task of having something collected from my door. I check the front door twice to make sure there is no one waiting there even though I have not heard a knock. I decide I better get the file out ready, so I spend a few minutes deciding where near the front door is the best place for it – the window sill, the stairs, the radiator shelf, the hat stand. I plump for the radiator shelf. Eventually the courier comes, knocks, Lucy answers the door and hands over the file effortlessly. I am lying on the floor in the playroom at the time having been floored, quite literally, by a series of other communications with the outside world.

First occupational health came back with an appointment time for next week – I emailed them after the first appointment last week. I had quite forgotten I was still waiting to hear from them. The problem they create is threefold, only one part of which is their fault. First it reminds me of the need to deal with the outside world. I have been nicely cocooned all morning in the home shell and suddenly I am reminded of journeys I have to make over the coming days and conversations I am going to have to have. Second (and this is their fault) they suggest a meeting on Tuesday 29th June which does not exist – it's Tuesday 28th or Wednesday 29th. And I have another appointment at 5.45 on the Tuesday – if I see occupational health at 4.30 will there be enough time?

Tears are now flowing down both cheeks and my hand starts to shake uncontrollably. Lucy calms me with a hand on mine and gets to work replying on my behalf. Later I see that she has had a whole exchange with the person concerned, made an appointment for the 29th and no doubt diarised it. Meanwhile I have lain on the floor (oh and watched some tennis).

Then I pick up a message on my mobile from my senior partner, Alan, asking very nicely how I am and saying that people are increasingly asking what is the matter, and that we need to agree some form of words. Now, you might think I could call him back and have the chat. He's a thoroughly decent chap, very sympathetic and kind. But no. Some tears to myself first. Then I need to talk to Lucy about it and we agree I will call him back and maybe suggest we meet – he lives round the corner. I have a fag first just to further delay and then spend a good minute scrolling all the way through my address list to ... A when, as luck would have it, Lucy tells me he has emailed her. I have been saved by the bell – no need to talk to anyone. Hurrah!

The whole thought of work and people there worrying about me and what we should be saying to them is too much though and I start crying. Lucy takes on the role of drafting a response while I lie *on the floor of the playroom crying (which is where I am when the courier arrives). I agree with whatever wording Lucy suggests and spend much of the rest of the day watching TV.*

So most of the day is spent sitting down, with small periods of limited exertion in between and three episodes of crying. But some small tasks are completed so that is a plus.

I watched a lot of sport on TV that summer. I have always wanted to do it but never gave myself the permission. There were always jobs that could be done, ways to be productive. In the back of my head there's also my dad's voice telling us to turn the TV off when we were young, because 'It's a lovely day and what are you doing wasting it sitting inside?' – my kids will have that voice from me now too. But now I was listening to my body more and giving myself the permission to do more of what I wanted to do, but also not to do more than I was capable of.

I also had the fortune of watching a day's play at Wimbledon, thanks to a friend of Lucy's whose father used to be a bigwig in the Lawn Tennis Association. It was hard to get excited about it. Illness seemed to take the edge off things – all my emotions were dulled somehow. And at the same time there was the anxiety of being in crowds.

Lucy looked after me as ever. I do not know what I am panicking about – the people, the space, getting lost, I just don't know but I start shaking and crying. I had a series of similar moments on the way home. The bus was okay then we went to Waitrose and I was rubbish in there, and again out on the street, and then again walking home and even just sitting at home – it might be over exertion. Also my legs were flaky. And I walked into things, twice cutting my legs on edges I had not seen. In one panicking moment I nearly lost my balance.

The issue of what should be said at work about my absence was a recurring theme. I was keen for people to be told what was wrong. Work were worried, I think, that colleagues and clients might be concerned about engaging with me in the future if they knew that I had had mental health problems. I understood where that concern comes from, and I was in no position to make a decision, but I am passionate now about the need for people to speak out about mental health. The reason why clients and colleagues might have had that reaction is precisely because of the silence and stigma surrounding mental illness. We will only break that down by talking about it. And when we do, as I continue to find, you realise just how many people you know who have had problems, or who know someone who has.

I also had moments of frustration. I was getting impatient that I was not getting medication – this was being delayed until the neurologist had completed his investigation lest any drugs reacted to any epilepsy I might have had. I also wanted answers as to how long this was all going to take ... How long am I going to be ill for? When you break your leg, they tell you x weeks in plaster and after y months you should all be fine. Why couldn't they tell me how long it took to heal a brain? Or at least how long was normal. There is, I know now, no normal, and no basis on which to make any such prediction.

I also got angry with being ill – why am I like this, why can't I be normal? Apparently, that's a pretty common theme. People ask, 'Depressed? What's he got to be depressed about?' It's annoying when others do that – it's an illness and I wouldn't ask someone what reason they had to be diabetic or whatever. It's particularly annoying and completely pointless when you are shouting those questions at yourself.

By the end of June, with a diagnosis beginning to firm up around depression and anxiety, I was signed off work for a month by the doctor, as opposed to the two-week periods he had done previously. It's double edged. On the one hand it takes away the worry of what is happening for the next month – nothing much. On the other, so it felt at the time (somewhat amusingly in hindsight), it was beginning to look like quite a long absence from work already. The longer it became, the huger the idea of going back seemed. And I knew from my employment law work the statistics that show quite markedly that once you get past a relatively short period of absence, the chances of ever going back start diminishing really fast.

Meanwhile, my relations with the outside world weren't getting any better. I could cope, sometimes, with seeing friends, as long as Lucy was there, promised to stay with me, and I was allowed to leave when I needed to. But the general public was another matter entirely.

Tuesday 28th June

Last night was very hot and I do not think I slept for more than an hour at a time, if that. It may have been the heat but may have been worry about the neurologist or other stuff. I feel quite apprehensive today. But ... I have a list of things to do. I am to visit the music shop to buy music for Gina and bits for the violin [despite lacking any musical ability we had decided it might be a good idea for me to try to learn to play something and, given the kids had done violin, we had plenty of books around to help me start]. *Then I am to visit Champion timber to get tacks to mend the laundry basket and go to Waitrose for food for a friend who is coming for lunch. I manage it all – but only just.*

People in music shops are just lovely. They seem to have all the time in the world. They appear to love their job and everyone they interact with while doing it. Visiting music shops should be a therapy in itself.

Waitrose, however, is a different matter. I find myself pushing and getting in the way of other people and having too many decisions to make – how am I supposed to know what to buy? I look at the list – tins of tomatoes I can manage, no real choices there. I opt for the value range on the basis that maybe we need to start saving money when we can – although we seem to be spending much less with me at home. Carrots are okay too. But potatoes? Which sort? How many? In the end I go for two different sorts but that takes a few minutes of standing staring. But that is the easy bit. Next the list says "lunch" and then "pudding". There is no "lunch" department and, even if there were, there would be no special sign saying, "Lunch for Richard to buy today".

So, I go round the entire shop to make sure I know all the things they sell before trying to make a decision, and then take 10 minutes to decide on some different tartlet things, some pots of salad and an apple tart.

Toothpaste next. For who? Which sort? Oh shit, there's a three-for-two on. Which brands? Do they all have to be the same? I am tempted to sit down and wait for someone to help me or throw me out. But eventually I manage to work out the rules.

After being seduced by various offers on familiar-looking items, and also priding myself on remembering we are running low on cereal, I head to the till. I am already worried because I did not bring any bags so am going to be shamed into using some from the store – 'Would you like a bag, sir?' – 'No, I think this will all fit nicely in my trouser pocket!' Of course I want a bloody bag. Which sort? Oh fuck. Anyway, as I approach the tills (ignoring the self-scanning tills because there is no chance whatsoever of me managing that and it will end up with someone having to do it for me) there are two tills with smiley ladies waiting to serve me, and no queues.

Now, that creates its own problem because I do not know which one to choose. As I am standing there frozen on the spot in a moment of some panic as to which one to go for, not one, but two ladies in Lycra push past me, one to each till – I am just not good at this game and am left mumbling to myself about how I thought I was next. Anyway, after a further moment of internal debate I start loading my stuff on to the conveyor belt behind one of them. Why are they in Lycra? I wonder. Have they been for a run, or is a trip round Waitrose their workout? It is certainly going to be enough for me.

As expected, I have the debate with the lady at the till about bags. I apologise for not having brought any. She offers me bags for life but we have enough of those to last the lifetimes of my great great grandchildren so I decline. Very kindly she opens the flimsy ones she passes me – I am not sure how I would cope with not being able to open them out myself. She gives me four. I say three will be plenty, I think and then have to spend a bit of time re-arranging to cram my goods into the three – for whose benefit was that, I wonder? The total is £61, despite the value range tomatoes. I came out for lunch for three and did not buy any booze – this saving money is not as easy as I thought.

Anyway, my great encounter with the world done for the morning, at least, I head home.

After unpacking and rejoicing in the accolades I receive for the lunch I have bought (although it seems I forgot the bread which was not on the list), I settle down to mend the laundry basket. This is not a big job but has the potential to go badly wrong. You might think I would take it to the shed but instead I opt to take all my tools to the cramped bathroom to do it there. Miraculously and despite all the risks, it works and by the end I have something that still looks like a laundry basket. A success and one that is rare these days, and very welcome as a result.

Lunch with Lucy's friend is very nice. She trained as a psychotherapist and then got diagnosed with bipolar and had major depression after a divorce, spending three months in the Priory, so we have a great time with Lucy, all exchanging depression stories. She is understanding, supportive, and kind.

The trip to London Bridge to see the neurologist looms. I look up the journey on the Transport for London travel planner – it says to take a train to Waterloo and then another from Waterloo East to London Bridge. I print off that part and look at the walk from there to the hospital which seems to be bang next door. Thinking even I can work that out, I foolishly decide to save the ink and not print the map. So, an hour later, I am cursing that decision as I wander for half an hour around London Bridge trying to find the hospital. At least I am giving myself 45 minutes of lost / panic time for these trips else I would be a wreck by now. Too frightened by the traffic noise, the building sites, the people, and the train noise, I dare not ask anyone for directions. After tears and several minutes of standing and staring, interspersed with pep talks to myself and bouts of confusion, I find myself in front of the hospital building, and behind me I see the exit from the station that I came out of 40 minutes ago.

Now, hospitals deal with sick people who must often be in a state of some disarray like me. So, how about we make them easy to find, welcoming when you get there, easy to navigate and put a kind person on the door. Or not. 'Sorry, sir, but you need to be in the building over there.' ' Where?' 'Over there.' 'Oh okay, sorry.' I find that building. 'You want the first floor, sir.' Okay – I turn to the lift as the doors close and I opt for the stairs. Reception is not called reception but something else. There are some sofas and a man says, 'Take a seat and I will call you in turn.' But there are loads of us waiting. How will he know the right order?

When called to a booth to check in, they want all sorts of information about me, my doctor, my BUPA number, postcodes, telephone numbers, authorisation numbers. Aha, but I have brought my new file that has all this information in it as long as I look hard enough. After completing it all on the computer and printing off two copies, one for me to keep, and one for me to give to the doctor, I then have to put all the same information on a handwritten form to give to the doctor. The man says he does not know why this particular neurologist insists on this. Perhaps it is designed to make life as difficult as possible for people who are ill and in an agitated state already as a result of their illness and the consultation about to happen. I begin to wish I was an inpatient so all this would be done for me and doctors would come to me and someone else would make decisions and appointments and stuff.

Eventually I get to see the neurologist. He has a spacious office overlooking the river. There are photos of his children. Proudly he tells me he has not read the referral letter. That makes me feel a whole lot better! So, I go through my history for the 83rd time in the last fortnight. I have been told that he is very good and definitely the expert I need to assess whether my funny turns are a form of epilepsy. So, when he starts looking things up on Google and Wikipedia, I am a little bit concerned. I am still not sure whether it was for my benefit or his. Anyway, we conclude that a lot of symptoms are in line with those of partial seizures. He wants to examine me physically so, as instructed, I go behind his screen to undress down to my boxer shorts, but then panic because I cannot remember what he said to do next. After a minute or two he asks if

I am ready, and, because he does not tell me off, I assume I have done the right thing by just sitting and waiting.

He does various things and concludes that it may well be epilepsy, but he wants to send me for further tests – an MRI and a sleep EEG. I pride myself on being able to ask him what the EEG will be like and how does the sleeping bit work. Apparently, I go in in the morning, they do a scan while I am awake and then leave me to go to sleep while they repeat it – so I start to worry about whether I will be able to go to sleep.

He says the possibility of epilepsy is good and bad news. If it is epilepsy, then the good news is that I have an answer and it can be controlled with drugs. The bad news is that I will not be able to drive until it has been controlled for a year. Great.

He fills in some forms, with the wrong Christian name it turns out, tells me I need to contact various different people to arrange the scans, have the scans, then go back to him. It all has to be just so – he wants this person to do the scan because they report in the way he likes etc. When I tell him the doctor has signed me off for a month he tells me he sees no reason for me not to be able to work. I tell him I cannot stop crying which seems to satisfy him.

The journey home is hell. I find the station okay, but am confused and totally overwhelmed by which platform etc. Meanwhile, I am in everyone's way as they rush home from work. A hen night group pass me all shouty and screamy. A pram runs in to me. I turn to apologise to the mum and bang in to someone else. I want to sit on the floor, close my eyes, and cry until they have all gone away. But that would not help. So, I ask someone which platform, and pigeon-step my way to platform six. Thankfully the train comes quickly and there is a seat for the short journey to Waterloo. The walk from there to the main concourse is just as bad. Even there on familiar territory I am scared witless and walk oh so slowly to the right place, sometimes stumbling, apologising to the countless people in whose busy way I put my directionless frame. As I find my train I start to panic because the early carriages are full and there are no seats. There is no way I can get to Wimbledon standing up.

Thankfully, the further carriages do have seats and I settle in the corner with my book and push the world away from me.

The evening is emotional. I feel much like the first week, and on the brink of tears.

CHAPTER 6

LEFT IN CHARGE
YOU CAN DO IT

As is probably quite apparent, in the weeks since my panic attack I had basically been looked after by Lucy. I made some day-to-day decisions about how I might spend the day, and even sometimes how I might spend the next day. But Lucy was actually taking care of everything that needed to happen, getting my help when I could give it, but making sure that what needed to be done was done. It was Lucy who ensured that the kids were organised and fed and clothed, that I did what I needed to do, that I went to where I needed to be, and was kept out of the way when I might upset people.

And the thing about mental illness is there are no rules, no one can tell you what you can and cannot manage, and when it's your first encounter with it, you have no experiences to fall back on.

For many months, long before I became ill, Lucy had planned a weekend away with some friends. We talked about it many times, whether she should go or not, and whether I could look after myself, let alone the kids. I wanted her to go. I did not want her to miss out, and she had more than earned the break. And maybe, somehow, we thought it might be a good test for me.

So, we managed to convince ourselves that it would be fine, that she should go.

Wednesday 29th June

I slept badly again. I am getting anxious about Lucy going away tomorrow. She has done me a schedule of what needs to happen each day, but I am acutely aware that until now I have barely needed to be responsible for myself and, although I can take responsibility when I want to and feel able to, when I can't, then Lucy takes over. For the next few days there is no one to take over and I am to be responsible, not just for me but for the kids too.

We have toyed with various different arrangements. The kids could all go and stay elsewhere but I am not sure I want to be on my own. I do not feel secure enough to be away from home and cannot face the prospect of someone else staying here with me with their own needs and their own energy, which will not allow me to withdraw – and I would end up feeling responsible for them which would not help. So Lucy has decided Jude will go and stay with Grandad and then Uncle Dick, and the girls will stay with me.

I keep re-reading the schedule. Nothing stays in my memory so my lack of recollection about what I need to do each day causes regular panics. I re-read the schedule again and again, but nothing sticks.

Thursday 30th June

I have another poor night's sleep, waking every hour at least. It may be the anxiety about Lucy being away. I log on to the Mind Gym website about CBT which looks interesting. They ask whether you are suffering different symptoms relating to depression and then anxiety. It turns out that neck pain and weeing a lot are anxiety-related symptoms. Well that explains a lot. The reality of Lucy being away is really dawning, but I try not to show my worry so as not to make her feel guilty. I know she would cancel if she thought I would not be okay, so I need to be strong. I drop her off at her friend's house – they are getting a taxi together to the airport – and say goodbye. And then I am on my own ...

I decide on supper. I also plan when it will happen and when I will cook. And when I go round to drop Gina at her violin lesson and the teacher says, 'Why don't you stay?' I agree first, then assert myself and say, 'No, I will go home and cook.' It seems a little thing but going along with what people want is easy; this was me taking control.

I lose my temper unnecessarily with Jude. I shake and then snap. It is uncontrollable. We are fine again afterwards but it scares him, me, and probably the girls.

I am feeling really quite vulnerable and alone. The next days are opening in front of me like a vast chasm. I want to have a drink to make it better but drinking on your own is frowned upon, but I think I am going to have to anyway.

Friday 1st July

It was only two glasses of wine in the end.

I slept really well but woke up feeling crap as always. I am tired and feeling like I cannot be bothered to do anything, and that I would struggle with anything anyway. I have nothing I have to do this morning, but I am anxious. I keep checking the schedule Lucy left me. What I need to do later is not that hard, but it feels a huge task ahead.

I need to take Gina to her violin exam then drop Jude at a friend's for her to take him to a cello concert, then go and pick up Steph and take her to the concert and then attend the concert. I decide we should drive past where the exam will be, just so we know for later. So, we drive and do not find it. We try again but still do not find it, so this increases the nerves. We go home and read the schedule again which says it is next to the fire station, which means the other direction entirely – so I have made myself worked up by not reading what I have been told.

Saturday 2nd July

A Get Well card arrived from work signed by all my team, which made me cry.

There is a street party down a road near us with people we know but I am not confident about going to that. I do not want to have to *talk to people and at the same time I am worried about being on my own. I do not think people want to talk to me and so do not want to be there. Also, the kids do not really fancy it either, so I use that as an excuse not to go. I arrange to go and see my parents instead, saying to people that I may come to the street party later, but I kind of know I won't.*

I sort out lunch – omelette using left over sausage – which was my own idea. It was not on the schedule and I did it without too much panic or worry, I think.

I am conscious I have not shaved or showered for several days. I need to take care of my appearance and personal hygiene but am failing badly.

All sorts of things started to make me feel guilty. Not washing was one. Another was buying a CD that I knew Lucy wouldn't like. I decided I wanted to buy a rose bower for the garden and became fixated about that and wanting to get it ready before Lucy got back so I could show how clever I had been and how I had coped. And I worried about having a card and cake and flowers to welcome her home, and how we had not spoken to her since she had been away.

In the meantime, we have a lovely Sunday, playing some tennis across the road, breakfast all together, a bike ride, some shopping – I had to leave one shop because the music was too loud and was making me anxious. And I emptied the ashtray in the garden which had been on my mind to do for several days – small things but well done, Daddy! It is important to recognise the things you achieve, however minor – we spend too much time worrying about the things we haven't done.

I am worrying that I need to do my diary and some work on the Mind Gym – why is that a worry? The CBT lady I am seeing tomorrow said quite specifically that it was entirely up to me and that it would not in any way impact upon treatment. So why has it become something I must do? I just cannot let it go. I feel guilty for not doing it, so I spend half an hour at it – I had already done some a couple of days ago as well.

Monday 4th July

It was an awful night's sleep. I could not get to sleep for hours. I went to bed happy, albeit that it was Monday the next day, but, when you do not have to go to work, Monday is less frightening. There is getting the children ready and some errands to run but really that should not be stressful, so I do not know why I was unable to sleep. I took ages to get to sleep then had that terrible waking up when it is still dark. You try to put off looking at the clock but eventually you do and there is that heart-aching moment when you see it is 4-something and you know that in the coming day you will be tired and drained.

I send an email to work to thank them for their card and the books they sent. Then some DVDs arrive too. They are box sets. It is really kind of them and I realise that Lucy and her brother Dick have been involved – when he dropped Jude off on Sunday I saw him glance at our pile of DVDs, presumably to make sure we did not have what he ordered. The problem is that I now worry about having to watch them all and when am I going to do it, because if I don't, it will look ungrateful, or they may think I did not want them and that will make them feel bad. And then I tell Lucy that on email and she admits her involvement and is sorry, and now I have upset her.

AAARRRRGGGGGGGHHHHH. Stop thinking like this.

Tuesday 5th July

Another awful night's sleep – booze makes no difference I can now confirm after two glasses of wine last night – and another demoralising glance at the alarm clock before 5.00am. It may be fear of what lies ahead, for today is MRI scan day. It is the first test of whether I am epileptic, and brings the promise of tunnels and loud noises and claustrophobia and, well, panic.

But I manage to get some things done this morning. I pick up an oboe book ordered last week and complete some other errands. It is a joy to revisit the music shop, an oasis of calm and trust and niceness. Back home I take a break, I notice how many light bulbs have gone but dismiss it with a shrug – it can wait. I have some lunch and watch a bit of TV before getting psyched up for the real business of the day.

Apparently, the hospital I am going to, although called King's and part of King's College, is known as something else for BUPA purposes. Helpful. Not.

My feet are heavy as I begin the walk to the station. Halfway there I wonder why I did not ride my bike, but it is too late now. I take the train to Waterloo, then another one to London Bridge, all going well. I know I need to head for Emblem House at London Bridge hospital. I get out and head for the exit. There is a sign to London Bridge hospital – Hooray, I think, and then remember I saw this last time and still got lost. But then I see another smaller one, taking me back into the station and over a footbridge – this is what I missed last time. Out of the window of the bridge I see the hospital and then Emblem House – get me, I have nailed it this time. A moment of elation and relief floods through me – small victories. I have 40 minutes to kill now – the time it took me getting lost last time – so I relax with an iced latte before checking in and being sent to the MRI unit.

There is a short wait while I fill in forms. Have I ever had operations? Yes a few. Ever had metal enter my body (e.g. a bullet)? No, I don't think so. Tattoos? No. Do I suffer from epilepsy? But hang on, that is why I am here having the damn test! The assistant and I agree a form of words to deal with that. Then I am called through and my heart starts to speed up.

I am shown to a locker to dump my stuff and remove all metal objects. The scanner is a giant magnet and so anything metal (except your wedding ring, I find out later) is sucked to the scanner – deeply lodged bullets can be pulled out of your body apparently. Then, in an outrageous attempt to confuse and distract me from the horror about to unfold, they ask what music I would like to listen to. They have a list and I opt for Norah Jones – soft, soothing, and something I haven't listened to for a few years.

I am asked to lie down on a bed on some sliding mechanism with the head end next to the scanner and my head is carefully positioned and then, without warning, a cage is fitted around my face and clipped into place. I am like Anthony Hopkins in Silence of the Lambs. No more than a couple of inches from my face is a cage which is clipped to the bed, so I cannot lift my head up. Responding to the terror in my eyes, the lady conducting the scan (who is perfectly lovely in all respects save for what she is doing to me) assures me that it is to get a better picture. She places my hands on my chest, and in my hand places a button to press if I am in any difficulty.

She then retires to another room and speaks to me through a microphone which comes through the earphones she placed on my head. I must have a microphone somewhere because she appears to hear me, although of course that might all be part of the act and, perhaps, I actually have no way of communicating with her. By now it is too late, and I am slid into the tunnel of the scanner and so, inches beyond the cage, which itself is inches from my face, is the wall of the scanner. Norah Jones pipes up, but after no more than a bar or two the scan starts with deafening, Doctor Who like, insane electronic noises coming from all around my head at a volume that completely drowns out poor Norah. It is like the death shrieks of a thousand Daleks and Cybermen as they fight a titanic battle to the death.

It is pure hell. I can feel the panic rising in me. The temptation to press the button is enormous. Then I think about the cage round my head, because even if they slide me out of the machine, I cannot escape – there will be a further delay before I can move freely and relieve the claustrophobia. So, I try to work out how long it would take to get the cage off and therefore how long do I need to leave myself between pressing the button and getting released before the panic breaks me, and how do I make that judgement?

I think of the irony of it all – I am here because of panic attacks originally and this is giving me the worst panic I can imagine. If you are not ill when you come in, you sure as hell will be when you leave.

I realise that I still have my wedding ring on and fear that will break the machine, invalidate the results or cause some other *problem meaning I have to go through it again. I toy with pressing the button, but I am thinking she will have realised by now surely.*

It is horrid, horrid, horrid. It is the worst torture I can imagine. I want to tell the kind lady every secret, betray all my friends and family, do whatever, if I can just get out of this.

After what seems an eternity, the noise stops. Norah is still going but I have missed the first few tracks on the album and I now remember why I stopped listening to it – after about track three the rest is God-awful. Then the sweet calm voice appears in my ear to ask if I am okay. 'Yes,' I whimper and then tell her I have my wedding ring on – 'No problem,' she assures me. What she means is that I am not getting out of it that easily.

'Halfway there,' she tells me and on we go to the next stage which is much like the first only with different sorts of noises – the Daleks are winning, I think, but have upped the power on their exterminator sticks to catch the fleeing Cybermen who are now in the next galaxy. After a further age of agony, it calms again. The nice lady comes on and says just one short 90-second set of noise to go now but, she warns me, it is louder and higher pitched and worse generally than before. I start counting as the sounds of hell begin. One, two, three, ... sixty, sixty-one, sixty-two, sixty-three and it stops. I have done it.

I am shaking as I am released from my imprisonment. The lights in the room are blinding on my eyes that have been held tight fast for more than half an hour.

I am a crying wreck as I emerge from the hospital. Tears are rolling down my cheeks, I am shaking, and once more I have to negotiate the journey back. Gone is the clear sense of direction and bravery of my arrival. Back firmly in place is the emotional incontinence of my last visit to these parts.

How I wish Lucy, or just someone, was with me.

CHAPTER 7

A NEW DESCENT

Although we were all still alive, and on the surface, nothing had gone wrong while Lucy was away, and I had therefore "coped", that impression was skin deep. I had been unnecessarily cross and short-fused with Jude, tense with all of the kids and, at the weekend, had managed to leave Gina waiting on the doorstep for 20 minutes, not hearing her knocking while I carried on mowing the back garden – aware in some strange way that she might be there but convincing myself she wasn't.

Lucy came back in the early hours of Wednesday morning. When she woke I suggested we go out for breakfast – I had already packed the kids off to school.

We go, and I order, and we sit outside. After a while I remember I need to tell Lucy that Gina had needed to put a story she wrote on a memory stick to take to school and we had found one that had some of Lucy's work on it, but we had checked there was space and sent this in with the story on a disc as well and a note saying the stick had to come home again that day. As I tell her this I break into tears, my body convulsing, my hands shaking. I can barely get the words out. She leads me gently home.

She tells me she is struggling to cope with me in this condition and is thinking I should go away, stay somewhere else, get admitted or something. She says I am also upsetting the kids. So here is an email I prepared to send to the psychiatrist:

Dear Doctor

I am thinking that I need to talk to you about the current plan.

I am really struggling day-to-day at the moment. Yesterday I had a major breakdown of tears and convulsions trying to tell my wife, Lucy, a simple issue about a memory stick. The day before I had the MRI scan which was a horrible experience. I have been keeping a diary over the last few weeks and I set out below the entries for the last couple of days which may help explain things – by way of context Lucy was away for a few days on a girls' trip planned months ago. Although not ideal timing, Lucy needed the break and we reckoned I would be okay, and largely I was, although we organised help with the kids. I feel like I have had a relapse since she got back.

So my mood is very variable.

For the record I have no suicidal thoughts or any thoughts of trying to harm myself. I firmly believe that I will improve and get to a better place at some stage.

I am really struggling to sleep at night and have never found sleeping in the day easy, and also have read that if I start sleeping in the day it is likely to further disrupt my night sleeping.

I take no joy in anything and the days are stretching out empty in front of me. I am doing things – see diary entries – but in small doses.

I think I need some medication to moderate my emotions and also to help me sleep. At the same time, I know that medication will take two weeks to take effect and that is despairing.

Lucy is struggling to cope with me as I am, having to cope with my emotional incontinence and would find it far easier if I was somewhere else. I do not think there is anyone I can stay with that can take me in, that I would be able to bear and who lives near enough for me to continue regular visits to London for treatment / tests.

It is also hard for the kids.

I also understand that until the neurologist has reported back to you on the possibility of epilepsy (which he seemed to think a distinct possibility), you are reluctant to prescribe medication. I have a sleep EEG booked for Wednesday next week, after which I need to see him and then you, which may be another fortnight. So, it is a month before any medication is going to take effect and I am not sure we can manage that as a family. We are also due to go away to France on 25 July.

So, the question is whether I ought to be admitted to hospital. The "benefits" are that it would give Lucy a break, would put me in the care of people who are used to dealing with people in my condition, would remove all responsibility from me (the need to contribute what I can to the running of the family and to limit the extent to which I am a burden on them) and might also speed up the testing process and therefore the onset of medication. It would also remove from me the trials of organising and getting to appointments with medics which can be very hard. (It would also remove the availability of alcohol which I am not taking to ridiculous excess, but am certainly taking – a few glasses of wine every night).

It carries some fears for me, but I suspect most of those are irrational.

So, what do you think? Does this make any sense? Ought we to talk or meet up? Would it help to involve Lucy? I think it would help me because I probably present a more together impression to professionals than is really the case because I am trying to be on my best behaviour! Lucy may be better able to tell the truth. Just writing this I feel tearful and hopeless – I can't even make a decision about what book to read next, and am intimidated by the pile of DVDs sent by work as a get well present.

Incidentally I had my first CBT session on Monday. It was largely a get to know you and planning exercise. The therapist is very nice, and I think we will work well together in due course. I have done some reading of stuff she gave me which all makes sense to me intellectually. I can see what it is saying okay, but I feel miles away from being able to do anything about it, I am too weak and unstable and am wondering, therefore, whether I ought to postpone further sessions until I am further down the track and perhaps medication has kicked in.

Please let me know your thoughts

Many thanks

We agreed that we would see how we were on Thursday morning before I sent the email off. Things were no better and so off it went. I don't know whether we had been pretending about how I was before Lucy went away in order to get us past that hurdle. Maybe the pressure of being in charge had pushed me over an edge. Perhaps Lucy had just been able to get some perspective while she was away to realise just how crap things were and maybe her friends had been able to give her some objectivity.

I was largely beyond having an opinion about what to do. I was scared about what was happening to me, was scared about the impact on our family, scared that I was on a downhill slope without any sense of where it ended. But I did not have any idea what to do about it and needed other people to tell me what was right. I had no trust in my own perspective, to the extent I had any perspective at all.

Thursday 7th July

Things start to happen, and they are being done without me. Lucy is talking to people and making plans and this is fine. I have withdrawn into my treacle cocoon again. I am back where I was weeks ago. I cannot feel the same person who was doing stuff only days ago. I shake, cry, and now sleep. I sleep for ages today. Was I keeping it all together for Lucy's trip and am I letting it all go? I feel like I am sinking. I sit doing nothing and thinking nothing and then the anxiety sweeps over me and I am inconsolable and quivering. I do not understand the link between the lawyer in charge of a department, to whom people direct their questions, who makes decisions about huge issues for clients, about people's careers, and the person I am now, who cannot make a decision for himself. How did it come to this?

The waves of panic are like physical pain. I am left gasping for breath, unable to bear it, but I do not know where the pain is coming from. I cannot just blame my leg or my hand or something. I cannot remove the pressure. I just have to breathe deeply and wait for the panic to pass.

What about the Priory? Getting admitted validates the way I have been – if anyone has doubted what I am feeling, then this surely will convince them. Who needs convincing? Maybe me, maybe my parents, I don't know. It will be a place of peace. All my worries will be taken away. Already I am relieved of the burden of worrying about anyone else and soon, even of worrying about myself. It will get me away from the kids, so they do not have to see me like this and worry, and will also give Lucy a break because she is finding it really hard. She walks the dog and cries for an hour.

When you are a parent, a grown-up, with the kids around, you are a legitimate target for questions, and for them to pass on to you the responsibility of making decisions. It is not unlike the office. Juniors come to me to ask my view all the time. Sometimes they need to. Often, however, they are just passing on the responsibility of making a decision. And so do the kids. What shall I cook, is it done yet, shall I lay the table, what drink shall we have, shall I have a shower, can I watch TV? If I am not there, they will decide. Because I am there, they want me to decide. So, until I am away from home I cannot be free from the questions, the responsibility.

After sleeping most of the day, we go by taxi to see the psychiatrist. He is kind and gentle. He asks me questions, and with Lucy there I do not have to pretend that I am capable or anything else. I sit on his sofa staring, or with my eyes closed. I cry most of the half-hour we are there. I defer to Lucy. I cannot talk above a whisper or a whimper so Lucy interprets for me. He re-states the history of tests etc., why, what, and when. I am with-it enough to fill in gaps. I understand it all and drift in and out of the conversation.

He asks if I want to be admitted. I do not know. I do not know whether I am someone who needs to be there – I don't want to be there under false pretences, or for people to wonder why I am there. I know I am barely functioning at home. So, we come to an understanding that I will be admitted if BUPA agree and he says he will talk to them, and I feel the burden of ring-mastering being lifted from me. Other people are taking charge. It is a relief, but at the same time scary in the sense that it is happening because I cannot take charge, and accepting that, obviously, is a stark acceptance of my own limitations.

We get home. I am less anxious. There is a plan. Others are in charge. Lucy is going to tell everyone. She worries that my family will think she is forcing me into this, or that it is her fault or something, so I will phone my mum tomorrow.

We have a last drink or two together. Then she takes me to bed and gives me a massage. She does not ask me if I want her to, she takes charge and just does it. I sleep like a baby. I wake at 7.00am with the alarm for the kids but Lucy gets up and I sleep again until 10.30.

Friday 8th July

So, it is all set, the approvals have been given and I am going to the Priory. I do worry. It says quite a lot about my condition, I think, but it seems the right thing to do. I pack my bag, not really knowing what to expect or what I will need – but clothes and a wash bag and something to read seem like a good start.

I have a number of panic moments en route. Somehow that feels right – validating the journey we are making.

Une Petite Pause – Early 2016

I am currently sitting in a café in a village in rural France. I have been staying in the French house for a few days. I needed to get away from life in London. I could feel anxiety building up in me and decided to get away. Having spent most of the week in the house, huddled by an open fire while the rain and wind took charge outside, today I have ventured out. I am surrounded by French men of a certain age and two ladies, one the café owner and the other an older lady sitting on her own. The men all know each other and when they come in they go round shaking hands with everyone in the place, except the odd bloke in the corner typing away on his laptop.

I just nipped outside the café for a fag – even in France you can't smoke indoors now – and on my way out ordered a café grand crème for when I came back in. Hmmm – a Coke is waiting on my table. I decide against trying to correct the error.

I have been writing this book now for a few weeks – on another level, I started many years ago. It's lonely on so many fronts. I am doing it on my own. Right now, I am living alone in France and being a foreigner exacerbates that sense of solitude. I am remembering and exploring my thoughts, feelings, and experiences of a few years ago which also turns my every thought inwards. Even though I think I am writing for an audience, for others to read, there is an ever-present question in my head whether anyone will in fact ever read any of this. Maybe I am really writing this for myself.

It is a strange feeling re-reading my diary from those years past and re-experiencing the feelings. They are very familiar and present on one level, but on another they seem a world away. The years since have changed me so it is strange to re-present those words from another age without re-framing them within my current understanding.

I fear I am stalling now, delaying telling you about my arrival at the Priory, while the French locals, just before 11.00am, are ordering their first cognacs. Meanwhile my laptop battery is beginning to run low, so I will leave them to it and exile myself back chez moi and get a cup of coffee.

But I can't go on yet. There is something holding me back which I need to explore. Writing this is creating a sense of dislocation which I don't understand, and which is not altogether comfortable. Physically I am dislocated here in France, away from friends and family and away from home, although this place hugs me in a way no other home can do. I have spent much of the week working but dislocated from those I work with. I felt that dislocation before I came here, and my solution was to reinforce that emotional sense of dislocation by a physical one.

When I reproduce and reflect upon my diary, I cannot escape the fact that it is me I am talking about. Not all the events recorded are familiar to me. In exploring it all, I feel drawn into it, and I am nervous about the exercise and worried about what I will find, or not find. If this is an exercise of trying to make sense of stuff, what if there is no sense to be found? And yet I do not feel able to avoid doing it. I have to do this, I have to delve into these memories, these images, these voices. I have put it off for several years but cannot ignore it any longer. Which all sounds like one of my funny turns, just spread over four and a half years as opposed to a few minutes.

I want to say that I feel discombobulated – partly I think because that's such a great word and we don't get the chance to use it nearly often enough. But it does not quite hit the mark – there is something about discombobulation (and you might need to say it out loud to get the point) that sounds fun, jokey. That's the bit that doesn't quite fit with how I feel.

CHAPTER 8

THE PRIORY

"The Priory" has entered our language as a place where celebrities go to deal with addiction. But when people talk about the Priory, they generally mean a hospital in Roehampton, on the edge of London, not far from where I live. That's not the one I went to purely because the psychiatrist I first saw, and who therefore took charge of me going forward, is based in another hospital. The Priory is in fact a group of many private hospitals dotted all over the place. They deal with mental illness in all its forms. Addiction is part of it, but they also deal with depression, anxiety, eating disorders, psychosis, bipolar disorder, and much, much more. The patients come from a wide background. Some are self-funding, some funded by private medical insurance (like me), and some are funded by the state.

One of the things I was most worried about before being admitted was what the other people would be like and whether I was ill enough to be there. My psychiatrist said the place was filled with people like me, and he was right. My overwhelming memory is that it was a safe place for me to be, where all the worries of the world were kept away, where I did not have to think about anything else but how I was and what was happening to me. And the people there were kind and every single one of them, staff or patient, seemed to know what it was like to face the void, to be broken and scared beyond words about whether, or how, you would ever be fixed. And, indeed, what being fixed meant, or even whether you wanted it.

To state the obvious, you meet and learn a lot about a range of different people, and in what follows I have made sure to preserve their anonymity and confidence. I was there for four weeks, and over that time people come and go. I stayed in touch with some for a while but over the years have lost touch. They were such an important part of my recovery and I am so hugely grateful to them all.

We shared of ourselves in a way I had never shared with anyone else, yet we began as strangers, brought together only by the common fact that we couldn't manage in the world. Together we got stronger. Given how close we became in many ways, the randomness of our meeting seems absurd – in a poem about a train journey, *The Whitsun Weddings*, Philip Larkin talks about his fellow passengers, "this frail travelling coincidence", which seems apt to describe our not so merry band. Had I been admitted four weeks later or earlier I would never have met any of them. But I would have met others and that, I guess, is the point. When you are broken, and you accept that sufficiently to reach out to strangers to ask for help, it doesn't really matter who they are, particularly if they need your help too, and each is happy to oblige.

At last we arrive. It's an old stately home set in parkland. Most of the parkland is public and there is a fence around the area closest to the building. We are welcomed warmly. Everyone is gentle and sincere. I am introduced to various staff whose names I forget instantly and, with Lucy still with me, am shown to my room by the admissions clerk. I shake and whimper quietly while Lucy unpacks for me. The room is pleasant enough, clean and smart with an en-suite bathroom. It is on the ground floor with a floor-to-ceiling sash window whose sashes open only a few inches, and, even then, there is a grill covering the small opening. It is to prevent escape I am later told.

At some stage Lucy must have left, after settling me in. I don't remember that. She had found me somewhere to be. I can only guess what was going through her head as she left me there.

There is a TV, but it does not work. This is because there are two different adult treatment programmes here, the general one and one for addicts, and the latter patients are not allowed TV, so they promise to sort that out, but I am not holding my breath.

I am on a half-hour observation cycle so someone knocks every 30 minutes to check I am still alive. I am also called on my room phone twice by an unintelligible voice saying something about medicine. I tell him on both occasions I am not allowed any, but I suspect he does not believe me.

As well as the two adult programmes, there is an adolescent group kept upstairs and quite separate from us adults. They have behavioural problems which explains the intense crashing and banging that strikes up mid-afternoon directly above my head, accompanied by a shower of debris falling outside my window. It upsets me but appears quite normal around here.

There is a directory of services to make it feel like a hotel, but it is really just a list of rules, mealtimes etc. I am not to have sex with other patients, drink alcohol, take or supply drugs, and must tell the nurse where I am. It's a bit like being at work.

The nurse arrives to take some details and check my belongings. He removes my razor lest I shave myself. I think he is meant to show me around but that will probably happen after the TV is fixed which will be after his shift is finished so may be some time. Then the doctor arrives and takes more details, many of them the same, so I am not sure who I have told what, but I give him the full monty, as much as I can.

I am surprised that they do not have my history. They clearly know some stuff but not everything.

Smoking is allowed outside in two wooden pergola things. I meet another patient there who asks if I have just "moved in" which sounds ominous. He moved in seven weeks ago and seems happy.

He shakes a lot – I wonder if that is more or less than when he arrived. He is on the general programme like me. He performs various impromptu magic tricks.

The food at dinner is nice and I eat with the nurse and the doctor. It is all quite informal.

Apart from the magician, I have not met any other inmates. There are 25 of us at the moment apparently – more will return after weekend leave. They all seem to know each other. I will need to make an effort to say hello and get to know them and it would be good to do that at the weekend while things are quieter, but I do not feel up to that now and will leave it for tomorrow.

No people, no TV, and no booze is a bit dull though ...

There is no plan for me as yet. I am told group sessions will happen on weekdays and I should use the weekend to settle in and forget all about worries from the outside world.

Saturday 9th July

I woke at six and read until getting up for breakfast – I had a shower and stuff, although no shaving of course. I psyched myself up to be brave and to approach people at breakfast to talk to them. I was knocking on the door of the dining hall at 7.45 but it did not open until 8. I went in with a lady and, having got breakfast, I ask the lady if I can join her.

She says no, that I am not allowed on her table because she is APT, the addicts programme, and they are not allowed to mix with us on the general programme. I feel completely deflated. The effort it had taken me to approach someone had been immense. I just needed to be with someone, to talk, to be accepted, to be human and have human interaction, and then it feels like I am rejected totally. I was crushed and ate with tears mixing in to my Fruit and Fibre. Someone else came in but sat at another table. I rushed my breakfast to get out of there as fast as I could. Later, as I read the papers outside, I could hear groups chatting happily to each other which just made my isolation worse. I think about packing and leaving. I think about calling Lucy but do not want to upset her and make her think she has (or we have) done the wrong thing.

I am wandering around about 10, in the process of phoning Lucy and asking to be taken home again, and someone says, 'Are you coming on the walk?' What walk? No one has told me. They point to the notice board and there it says 10 o'clock group walk. I had no idea but jump at the opportunity to spend some time with people. It is great. We wander slowly, feed the ducks, a bit like children. For our little group Daddy nurse has brought the bread and he asks me if I would like to help them feed the ducks – not do it myself you understand, that might be too much, but help them. I am a child.

That simple moment finally brought home to me the state I was in. The reason why I was being treated like a very small child was because that was how I was presenting to the world. These skilled and kind carers were not reducing me to that state but rather responding to it, and if that was what I was like then I had better accept it and go with it … The 30-minute checks, the rules about not leaving the house without saying where I was going, the non-opening windows, the confiscation of my razor – they weren't there to protect the hospital, but to protect me. I really was that dangerous – to myself, I ought to make clear, not to other people. All the protections we put around our children when they are little were being put around me and in a quiet, shaky, scared little voice, I said okay – please will you look after me because I can't do it myself.

After the walk we sit down with a nurse who wants to plan some activities and we end up going into a room for a "group session".

I ask again about my TV and am told it will be Monday before they can do anything. I mention the noise from yesterday and ask if I can move room. It sounds like this is something that could be done but does not seem like it is something that will be done. It does not seem like action really happens here. There is a slow pace to life.

[Later on] *Oh how my world has changed. I have my orientation tour to show me around, and mention the room change again and it has happened. And I have a group of friends who introduce me to others. I feel settled in and calm and relaxed now. I have not had* tears and anxiety since this morning. This morning I had been toing and froing in my head about whether to tell Lucy how bad I was feeling. I did not want to scare or worry her. But I felt I had to talk to someone and I was literally dialling and the phone ringing when someone asked me about the walk and suddenly things started to improve.

The stories of my fellow patients are scary. Outside you ask people what they do or where they live. In here you ask what they are in for. There are attempted suicides of different sorts, or at least overdoses, and it is scary how easily it can happen. I hear the expression 'I had to do something to make people notice me, make them realise I was struggling.' It makes me think about all the times I have thought about how harming myself might make people realise I cannot cope, that it wasn't actually all okay, and might give me a chance to step out of the rat race. Why did I never feel able to tell anyone? Why did I never take those moments of despair seriously? And what stopped me following through with the thoughts?

What strikes me is how supportive people are to each other here – whatever pain they are going through, they are able to reach out to other people and talk to them and ask how they are and encourage them and welcome them. It is an extraordinary community where, within moments of meeting someone for the first time, you are in deep discussions about why they tried to take their own life, or their relationship with their father or wife, or whatever.

Big D has bipolar and has been on a shopping spree. He is very open about it. Recently he has bought a Scottish island. Today he has bought a dongle, a pair of shorts, and three pairs of trainers, because they were cheap. Apparently, shopping is a common symptom in the high periods of a bipolar cycle.

I am worried about Lucy visiting tomorrow. I do not want her to feel she has to because I am in despair or anything. I am also a bit scared of seeing her. It feels like the outside world raising its head to wobble my newfound calmness. We speak on the phone and agree she will come on her own without the kids and that seems best. It will be lovely to see her I think, but it will make me cry.

Late evening, I am outside the back having a smoke slightly out of sight when the door crashes open and two kids from upstairs come racing out – an escape attempt – how exciting. The house alarms go off. I do not intervene because I do not know whether to or how, and I am not responsible.

Earlier I overheard a discussion which makes you realise where you are. The magician was on a sofa in a public area working, and then called a nurse over to ask if the nurse could get the doctor. The doctor came and the magician asked if he could go to town to buy some fags and something else. There was then a 30-minute debate about it. The consultant was called and all sorts. You see, of course, as the doctor says, there are two sides to it, one being the magician just wants some fags which the staff could just as easily get him. The other side is the magician having an encounter with the world, which he is now being encouraged to do, and he has come up with this proposal as to how, when, and why, and it is a big issue. He was asked how he feels about going into town. And in here that question is valid and fair, and gets a sensible polite answer because how we feel is all that matters.

Sunday 10th July

I chat to some fellow patients over breakfast. The rest of the morning is bad. I am scared and anxious and shaking and tired. I worry about what I am doing here and all this time that is going by with me here. I find it hard to concentrate. At the end of conversations this morning I was struggling to finish sentences. I know the word I want and what I am trying to say, I just can't say it so there are pauses. I am close to tears. I sleep for some time but am awoken by the cleaner. Everything is heavy, heavy, heavy. I am worried about Lucy coming. What will we do, and what will she think, and am I allowed out, and am I trying hard enough, and why do I keep shaking? Gone completely is the confidence of yesterday. I can't breathe. I want to scream and shake. I am not alright. I need to find again the peace and tranquillity.

[Later] *It was great to see and hold Lucy. We talked and walked. But I felt when she was here that I could collapse into her, maybe.*

I did not want to make her worry about how I was coping, but I still ended up wobbly, vulnerable, and a bit tearful. She left after a couple of hours and I went to sleep. I was glad that she had not brought the kids because they would have needed attention I could not give them. When Lucy told me what they were doing or the things that were happening, plans, schedules, I just zoned out, else I would have been overwhelmed with panic. I can live in the here-and-now but any thoughts of plans, of things that need to happen, of places I need to go, or anything complex, and I begin to panic.

It is immensely hard for those that love people who are mentally ill. Our natural instincts are all about helping, caring, resolving, making things better. And they can't. All they can do is be there when you need them and listen when you want to talk. And that is enough, that's all we need. There is no need to tell us what's happening in the world, unless we really need to know, because we can't process it and we can't engage. We are too busy with the chaos, the breakdown, in our heads. Sometimes you walk past one of those boxes in the road where telephone wires and internet cables are connected, and you see the mass of wires that make no sense but clearly are connected in some order. Imagine they weren't. If who we are (or who people take us to be) is based on how we respond and think, then basically the person you know and love is not there, or not all there, because all those wires have melted or been ripped out and scattered.

It takes time and space and permission to let the person find sense again themselves, and only they can do it. They may need help but that is probably best coming from a third party, a professional. The most you can do, in fact the best thing you can do, is show them you still love them and ask them every now and then how they are, but be prepared for the answer not being what you are used to or hoping for, and don't expect it to make a whole lot of sense to you. And you do not need to provide answers or solutions, or even make suggestions. Very often they will be beyond us and make us worse. Just listen and try to understand.

I awoke to one of my fellow patients calling me. Her husband had left after visiting her and she did not want to be alone, so we walked in the park and had an ice cream. We saw someone who I think is a partner from my work and we scuttled off. I did not want to have to talk to him and explain what I was doing in his local park.

While I was sitting outside later, a family drew up in their car. They looked like they wanted the park, but they read the various hospital signs and hurried off nervously.

Monday 11th July

The place has been buzzing today, at least in comparison to the weekend. Loads of consultants and therapists, new patients, lots of outpatients. It is a different world.

I was a bit anxious that I did not have a care plan and so did not know what I was to be doing and also that I did not know when I would see the consultant or meet my special therapist who would determine my plan and the groups I should attend. Anyway, the psychiatrist found me before sessions started and we had a chat which was fine, just a check-up really. He reassured me.

Then I was told to go to group support. We all sat in a circle and introduced ourselves, apart from the last person who did not feel like talking. Then conversation flowed which was interesting – exchanging experiences, how we felt, and also responding and commenting on what others said and felt. I cried a few times. Then I was sent to a CBT group session on avoidance which I do not really get. I had to ask what they were talking about a couple of times. I could sit and say nothing, but it is clear that the medics here think this therapy works and so if I am going to be here, which I am, then I might as well throw myself into it and participate as fully as I can. And make sure I know what is going on.

After lunch I meet my therapist. We go through my history again – the 500th time it seems. Then we look at the diary of group sessions and she makes a big play of choosing the right ones for me to do which, bearing in mind I am not an addict, am a bloke (which rules out the women's psychotherapy group) and do not have anger issues, is not that tricky.

Then yoga, which is a first for me and seems okay – if only the bloke lying next to me did not stink so much – I keep being told to breathe deeply but when I do I get two full lungs of unwashed, stale feet, groin and armpit which makes me want to vomit, so I find myself holding my breath which apparently is not right.

Big successes for today:

- *One of the group had a bath and got dressed. What I mean is not that it was a great success that at least one of us bothered, but that there was someone who hadn't for a while – and today she did.*
- *I got involved in the programme.*
- *I went into town and managed fine – I wanted to get some water and also check out whether I might feel able to get to the Tube in order to visit home at some later stage and that was okay.*
- *I spoke to some new people.*
- *I had a nice call with Lucy, but I cannot deal with all the arrangements and everything at home, and hearing her going through everything, and all the house noise in the background, was really too much and was making me panic. I have texted her to say as much and I hope she understands. I know she is having to shoulder everything, but I feel the need to protect myself here.*

I am really lucky that this is all being funded by work insurance and that they are paying me in full – I cannot imagine how we would be coping if we had to pay for this and my salary had stopped – I would not be here, I know that, and I would probably have forced myself back to work which would have been awful.

There is mayhem tonight. The darlings upstairs are running riot, setting off the fire alarms three or four times already and it is only 10.00pm. The addiction people are shouting at the staff because they want to make phone calls or something, and want to leave the door open to get back in after smoking. But the door has to be shut due to the kids kicking off, and the staff have their hands full and cannot deal with calls, and no one is communicating or listening or trying to understand each other – so much for all the therapy round here. How do you feel about this?!

75

Tuesday 12th July

I do sometimes question whether I should be here. There are loads of people far worse than I am. Sometimes I walk past a room and see someone inside who has not been out of their room all the time I have been here, so they must be in a bad way. I know that I was in a bad state when I came in but, even so, I am certainly at the mild end of the range of issues and am the only one I have spoken to who is not on medication, not yet at least. I am the only one who cries in all the sessions though.

But I am here, and the psychiatrist decided I should be. Comparison with others makes no sense. If it is helping me to be here, then it is good that I am.

I had two great sessions today. The first was psychodrama. We began with some breathing exercises then did some group work. The best bit was the acting out of dramas. Two people came forward to say they wanted to play stuff out. The first had two voices in his head, one saying he was weak and could not do anything and it was not worth trying as he would be bound to fail, and the other being firm, saying pull yourself together, get on with it, stop being weak and lazy.

He had to flip from one to the other while they argued with each other and someone else was asked to stand in for him on the other side of the conversation. He played out how these voices viewed and spoke to each other. Eventually the weaker one persuaded the firmer one to listen and they ended trying to support each other, but it was highly dramatic. Two things stay with me: one the fear that prevented each from trying to understand and reach out to the other, although the fear was stronger in the firm one, and the other was that it was somehow reflective of the conversations Lucy and I have.

The second volunteer was playing out her role within her family, presenting what she thought, but then she had to take the role of her father, then her mother and her sister, and talk to herself as if she were them. Again, it was fascinating looking at the different perspectives.

In the afternoon, we did mindfulness which seems to be all about focusing on the here-and-now, living in the moment (as opposed to for the moment) and making sure you experience fully the now. I did find real peace in meditation. We did an exercise of imagining you are in a cinema and you are projecting your thoughts onto the screen. Then try to go to the back seats to create a gap between you and your thoughts – so often we associate ourselves with our thoughts, as if they were us. But they are just thoughts and we can create that distance if we can learn to observe them.

Other successes today? I talked to some new people. I have got my head round going to King's for the EEG tomorrow, and I persuaded one of my fellow patients to come along to the mindfulness session.

CHAPTER 9

MEN CAN TALK
ABOUT HOW THEY FEEL

Wednesday 13th July

Today is EEG day. Before that I had two sessions this morning. The first was a men's support group which was good – a different dynamic to the mixed group support and useful, although a bit melancholy. There was a common theme of facing a work environment that was too obsessed with money. The second was a self-awareness group which focused on talking about how we felt.

When I first saw a men's support group in the timetable, I did wonder whether it could really work, whether a bunch of men really would talk and, if so, what about? But it turned out to be a real highlight of my time at the Priory. We talked about how we were and how we felt. We supported each other, and we were men – what it said on the tin.

The ever-changing population meant that there were guys who had been around for several weeks who set the tone and created the environment in which the rest of us felt able to talk, felt that we had permission. There were no alpha males using their sense of power or insecurity to direct the conversation. Our backgrounds were diverse, as were our ages. There were at least a couple in the group who were older than me, one or two of a similar age and quite a few who were younger – late twenties and thirties.

It is a truism that men do not talk about how they feel. They rarely talk to their partners about it, and certainly don't discuss it among other men. Our upbringing, societal stereotypes, the role modelling on TV and in the media do not encourage men to explore their emotions with themselves or their mates. I often feel that there is a competition going on when men meet. At work it is about who is more successful, more hard-working, next in line for promotion. In that environment you are not going to talk about feeling scared, or in doubt. You have to be driven and determined.

In other environments the competition may be about material wealth. I have listened (because I can't and won't compete) to conversations about the cost of the bikes they ride and the lengths they went to in order to acquire them, the amount their wives spend on whatever, the value of their house – or about who is funnier or more knowledgeable, or how successful our kids are at this or that, and how many activities they get involved in. The competition is not explicit but always seems to be there under the surface, and not too far beneath it either.

Here we were equal, brought to a level by virtue of our illness, and shorn of who or what we were in the world outside. As the discussions unfolded I realised how much we had in common, how the feelings and experiences and fears that I had were the same as others. At first, I listened and heard my voice in theirs and gradually that gave me the confidence to know that my voice too was valid and would help others in being heard.

As with every group session, we would begin with a check-in – going round the group in turn with everyone being asked to say how they feel right now, what is on their mind, what they would like to get out of the meeting. It is such a simple exercise but so powerful. As an individual you are forced to reflect on what you are feeling, rather than on other people and how they are. You get to know how everyone else is, who is in need, and how you can expect people to be during the course of the meeting.

So often in work or elsewhere, we have meetings where we have no regard to how people are. We have an agenda of business items to cover and expect people to contribute as if they were automatons. I never did get back to the team I led in my law firm, but I had in mind that when I did, our fortnightly meetings would begin with just that – how are we all, what is happening for each of us, and how can the team help. Plainly I would not expect people in work to bare their souls in front of all their colleagues, but it is clearly important to have a sense of how your team is doing, and, as a leader, if you listen sensitively and non-judgementally, you may pick up the signals that someone needs to talk "off line". At the very least we can ask, 'What do I need to know about you today?'

A while ago, I was delivering some mental health awareness training to the legal team in a global organisation. We began with a pilot session in London for some of the most senior members of the team from around the world. They were mostly, but not exclusively, men and, although all senior, some were definitely more senior than others. Once I had set the tone for what we were discussing, and talked about what anxiety looks like and some of the risk factors for depression and anxiety, I asked them what work life was like for them. I had allowed 20 minutes or so for that part of the session. It went on for at least twice that.

When people at different levels heard each other talk about the anxieties they felt, about the pressures and demands, and realised that they were all experiencing the same things, and were able to talk about it, they saw each other and their experiences in a new light. They wouldn't stop. I am not going to pretend that any of the demands, pressures, and anxieties went away or were solved that morning, but being able to talk to each other about them made a huge difference.

So many of my interactions now begin with the question, 'How are you?', and I hope people understand that I want to know the answer.

Yesterday I was sitting outside looking at the ground and noticed how grass that had been walked on gradually sprang back up. I could see individual stalks stand back up again. Some did it from their own strength, some helped by the wind and some the sun, and I thought that was how I might be – trampled – although not sure I feel the springing up again yet. Maybe I just need to find some wind and sun.

In the self-awareness group we were asked to go outside and find things that represented how we felt. So I found a bright yellow flower, small and delicate that seemed to reflect that we are all beautiful people, although feeling very small. It had been bent over by the wind so its stalk was at a right angle describing how we have been bent and burdened by our troubles. It danced around as it was buffeted by the breeze and moved according to how it was blown by life's difficulties. But, until I picked it, it was rooted, however lightly, to the ground, but firmly enough to keep it anchored which is how I feel. I am not without hope.

Then I found a stick that's about 10 inches long, strong and aged and weathered. It is curved as it had clearly been blown by the wind in its formation and had moulded itself to its experiences and surroundings. But it had been picked clean, stripped of all its bark in a way that looked deliberate, determined and complete, something that could only have been done by a person. That felt like me.

When meditating I had an image of being on a beach, the tide rolling in and out, in time with my breathing. I could imagine building a sand castle of all my worries and concerns – simple or hugely intricate – and then watching as the tide, my breath, gradually washed them away and left a flat, clean, expanse of sand.

So what about the EEG? The journey there was largely fine. Lucy arrived mid-test. They let me know she had arrived just before I went to sleep which was comforting, and afterwards we had a lovely drink and snacks at the station bar.

The test itself is nothing to fear. They give you some sleeping pills and attach electrodes all over your head. Then you lie down and they monitor you as you open and close your eyes to order and answer questions. Then there is a slightly nasty bit while they put flashing lights in your face at various frequencies. One made me shake a bit. Then they let you fall asleep – there is a bit of pressure to fall asleep, but the drugs worked. Then you get woken up which is a bit of a shame as you have just got cosy. A bit woozy and then back to normal. I have to wait for the results, but it feels like a step forward.

It was so nice to see Lucy, so comforting to know she had arrived and then wonderful to see and hold her, and we had a great chilled time afterwards.

CHAPTER 10

UPS AND DOWNS, AND MOVING ON

The next couple of days were a bit flat. I was conscious of people I had grown close to leaving, and towards the weekend there was an end-of-term feel about the place, all talk about plans for the weekend, the summer, going home. I did finally get medication. There was still no verdict from the neurologist so I guess it was a bit of a risk, in order to put me out of my anxious misery. Even though they would take a couple of weeks to start taking effect, the fact I was taking them was a relief and almost a boost in itself. I had a good CBT session thinking about the rules, the understandings of the world, that we pick up and stick to.

I was allowed home for some of the weekend. The kids were away, so it was just me and Lucy. She was wary about me coming because she was suffering a bit herself and did not want the added burden of looking after me. I popped in to a newsagent on the way back and then panicked when I saw someone I knew and hid to avoid having to talk to him – I had not thought about the possibility of seeing other people.

We had a good time on Saturday, and went out for dinner in the evening. I made a point of facing out of the window to avoid the view of, and the resulting anxiety caused by, the other people. Sunday was very subdued. There was a feeling of waiting to leave. Lucy was tired and went back to bed, so I ended up packing my bags and setting off back to hospital mid-afternoon. It was a relief to get back in a way.

Monday involved a range of sessions including something called behavioural activation where we set simple goals, for the short-, medium- and long-term, the idea being we can carry them round with us and take them out every now and then to chew over and then put them away again. My short-term goal was getting the report from the neurologist which was coming the following day.

Tuesday 19th July

It is the early hours and I am awake again. It is still dark. There is no hint of dawn behind my curtains which open onto a small grassed courtyard area surrounded by other rooms. The bathroom door is open and through the crack I can see the iridescent orange lights from the bath and shower controls, touch sensitive for some reason I cannot fathom. They emit a constant reminder of the regime of the day to come.

In my room there is the pale glow from my BlackBerry beside my bed, ready to sound the alarm at 7.10. And high on the wall opposite my bed is a blinking green light from what I assume must be the fire alarm. I am alone in the stillness of the night with only these lights as company. I am confused. I awoke first hours ago and checked the time, four o'clock it seemed to say. I know I was awake for a long time after that and now as I check again it still says four o'clock. My BlackBerry has not stopped. They do not do that.

I realise with a sinking heart and head that I first awoke at 12.20, that I must have had less than an hour asleep before that, and that between then and now I have slept only briefly.

I do not feel anxious or agitated. I do not know why I have woken like this. Sure I am getting the neurological results today but they will be what they will be, I just want to know the score. What is worrying me now, however, is the lack of sleep and I try all manner of different positions and thought processes to cajole my tired head back to sleep. I toss and turn for what seems an age, alone in this sleepless night. In the end, the alarm does wake me, so I must have drifted off to sleep again at some stage, but I feel none of the vigour and energy that sleep should bring. It will be a long day and with it, perhaps, much emotion as my body lacks the strength to control my feelings and my tears.

I went to see the neurologist and ... I do not have epilepsy. Just writing those words is fantastic. It is such a relief, such a weight off my mind. I had rationalised things either way, ruminating behind the closed doors of my mind, about the possible outcomes and now I know there is nothing to worry about. There is some deep infection of the synapses or something and some mild damage, possibly from an earlier head injury (maybe rugby or something), but otherwise all clear.

It does not explain the seizures but maybe they are a form of anxiety attack and, not having listened to them in France, my body gave me a great big shot of panic attack to make its message as clear as can be.

It was lovely to see Lucy at the hospital and catch up, and great to get a text from the kids. I sent home some cookies with Lucy.

I had reflected earlier that I had spent the last several months, and possibly years, at work in a state of semi-crisis or panic, always with a million things to worry about, to plan, to cajole people about, and implement. That really has to change somehow. That is going to a big task but not one for today, or, indeed, tomorrow.

That sense of having been in a state of panic for years was a real eye opener. I had not paid any attention to how I felt really, but now I could look back and realise that was how it had felt. I see that in some of the people I work with now, noting the way they seem to be, and asking whether they are aware of that and okay with it. The answer is generally that they cannot see any other way of being, which is so sad to hear, but I hope they do reflect at some stage and take the ownership of it that only they can.

Wednesday 20th July

I feel like a new man, that I have made huge progress over the last day or so. I saw the psychiatrist first thing and we talked for the first time about me being discharged, about plans for the weekend and about holiday. He sees that I have made much progress. My short-term aim was to get a diagnosis which I have now, albeit one that excludes epilepsy, rather than explaining the funny turns, but that is enough. Sometimes that is the most medicine can do. My medium-term goal was to be well enough to return home and be able to work towards the future. So, I will go home on Friday night and come back on Sunday. I will have the kids around and maybe try to see some other people.

I talked to my key worker this afternoon about strategies to deal with the kids and some of the dynamics that might arise. I shall try to make time to be with each of them on their own, somewhere safe, to reassure them about my progress. I also need to make sure I have some time on my own to chill out and that we keep some flexibility. I am really looking forward to it. Then we can review how it all went on Monday and, if okay, discharge me next week. I can come back for some sessions as a day patient and then go on holiday in August.

It feels so nice to have a plan, to have some certainty, to look beyond the next day or so. I have been deliberately living day-to-day, taking each day as it comes, but to be able to lift my head a little to look to a more distant horizon is a great privilege. I will be better, and it is happening now, or at least beginning to happen. It may not be the beginning of the end, but it feels like it may just be the end of the beginning.

I continue to connect with people and feel that people value me and that I am a help to them. That is important to me. In self-awareness we looked at who we feel emotionally attached to and put them in orbits around ourselves, and right now a number of the people here feature much more closely than many of my friends and family. That is in part because I am in lockdown here, I have deliberately not sought to communicate with people outside and have discouraged them from communicating with me. That has put the burden on Lucy, but it has been important to give me space and not to have to explain and validate myself to everyone. It is a safe, calm, and kind place to do that.

At the same time the dynamics of the inpatient group are changing. The people who were here when I arrived are slowly moving on and being replaced by people I seem to connect with less easily – that is probably more about where I am now and my thoughts turning to leaving than anything about them. It is not always easy to believe the stories they tell me, and it is hard to know what to do or say in response. For some there seems to be a desire to seek status through their stories, competing with each other to out-dramatise their experiences, while at the same time not wanting to focus on how they can help themselves.

I was called the most sane-looking person one can imagine today, which must mean I am making some progress and the reaction from everyone to my test results has been lovely. People were genuinely happy for me. It was very touching.

[Later] Sadly it looks like there may have been a suicide from the hospital. A group member's brother is a fireman and called him to say there had been a call out to a suicide under the tracks at Southgate Tube station and there are police here this evening, and the hospital director is here which is odd for the evening. I just hope and pray it is not the case. Thinking about it, I had noticed the air ambulance was circling for a long time this afternoon, looking for somewhere to land.

Thursday 21st July

Unfortunately, I was right. I overheard conversations at breakfast which seemed to suggest that was the case, but we received the news mid-morning that it was one of the people who had been around for some time. A quiet, kind, and dignified man. We do not know the cause of death for certain, but the assumption is suicide. It was his last day as a day patient. It looks like he walked out of his last class and went to the Tube station and then it happened.

The news, of course, hangs over the whole community. There is deep shock, a lot of speculation and I am guessing a lot of discussion among the staff as to whether they missed anything. For some it is evoking memories of their own previous attempts at suicide, or those of people they know. People say it is such a hard, big decision to make. But to me it seems a desperately simple decision to make, if that is what he did – it could have been the spur of the moment without time to think – the opportunity was there suddenly and that was it. It may not even have been intended.

One of the striking things about mental illness is the matter of fact way in which suicide is discussed. It is one of the first questions that any professional will ask you about – have you had suicidal thoughts and, if so, have you given any thought as to how and made any plans? At first it seems very strange, but you soon realise that it is a matter of risk assessment first and foremost – what are we dealing with here? And the fact that you are confronted with it in such stark terms forces you to ask the question of yourself. All the research shows that it is a good thing to do, and, contrary to some myths, it does not put a thought of suicide into people's minds that was not there already. The chances are that if you are ill enough to have the question asked of you, the thought of suicide will have occurred to you on a number of occasions already at some level. After a while it becomes a form of self-check almost. Yes I am feeling anxious, yes I am feeling low, yes I have thought about suicide, and while I might have thought about how I might go about it, I have not made any detailed preparations.

We had a session this afternoon on relapse prevention which talked about the cycle of depression – you have a low mood so you stop doing things, including things that normally lift your mood, so that this creates a lower mood and so you stop doing even more things. The idea is to break the cycle by forcing yourself, through scheduling, to do something that you have not been doing. It might be a chore or it might be fun, but schedule time to do it, and stick to the schedule.

The context is you drop hobbies and other things, seeing people and the like, leaving you only with work and chores and then they become too much. I wonder whether in fact I have been depressed for ages and just not realised it – whether I am in some way immune to mood or have such a low expectation of mood that I just go along with low mood and do not reflect on it. I do not see my friends. I do not keep up with hobbies. I convince myself there is no time and I do not deserve them.

Friday, Saturday, and Sunday
I am writing this on Sunday evening back at the Priory.

Going home was wonderful. I so enjoyed seeing the children, feeling the warmth of their hugs, the intensity of their having missed me, and me them. Lucy, however, seems distant. We hugged and she seemed pleased to see me and hear that I was doing well. But she seems very low. She slept a lot and when awake was often distracted, focusing on the chores and the email inbox. There is a tension around the amount of time and care I am getting – 'What about me?' she seems to be saying. I know it is hard and I know she needs support and love, she needs to be looked after herself and is at the end of her tether looking after everyone else. She also wants to move on from where we are, to make decisions, to make change.

On Saturday we went for a bike ride to the common and then went to see a house she thinks we might want to buy, to downsize, get rid of the mortgage and release the pressure. The house is smaller and the garden is smaller, but it won't be cheap enough to pay off the mortgage. I do not like it and I feel I am disappointing her. I do not feel ready to agree a move in any event. If I tell her, however, I fear she may get down because she has invested her time and energy, and may feel she has done the wrong thing in suggesting it. But I never said to go ahead and start looking. It feels like she is just running ahead when I am barely able to walk. I have to stay in the moment for now and take each day as it comes. Big decisions will need to be made in due course, but not now.

After viewing the house, we cycled on. One of the kids began telling a strange story about a comfy chair that had been left in a shopping trolley beside the road and it set off some kind of déjà vu in my head, quite momentary that did not lead on to a funny turn but felt very like the beginnings of one. I stopped, recognised it for what it was, and then moved on. Later I felt quite anxious and when we got home I was exhausted and slept for two hours.

On Friday, I went to Waitrose to conquer some demons, and bought a bottle of Champagne. It turned out to be corked so Lucy returned it on Saturday, getting a double refund which paid for supper and some Prosecco, and some biscuits for the kids. I also went to the chippy and made decisions about what to buy. It was busy in there and I held it together.

On Saturday I phoned Mum, but did not speak to various other people who had been in touch and who I had half planned to call. I emailed work to update them, and also thanked a couple of partners for their cards / letters.

Coming back here this evening felt like a regression. It was nice to see some people, but others seem to still be finishing off the same sentences from Friday, the same issues, going round and round and round. I feel separated from them, like I no longer fit in. I do not have the patience to hear it when it is going nowhere – it is talking for talking's sake without thinking or listening and without a desire to do anything with or about it.

Monday 2th July

I completed a mindfulness body scan this morning. I had done one the other day lying down on the grass outside but found my attention drawn more to the ants crawling up my shorts than the rhythms of my breathing! This time I tried it lying on my bed so rather fewer bugs to disturb me – it was good. I went for a coffee and had a shave, so it was a busy morning before classes. I had various classes which were fine and then a good session with my key worker who was helpful, and we agreed that I need to find a way to get Lucy some help of the kind I have been getting here. We talked about what I would do as an outpatient, the classes I would attend, and then what I would do on days off.

And then I saw the psychiatrist who is happy with the idea that I am ready to go home and that, in fact, staying is likely to hold me back. Hurrah! So the plan is to go home tomorrow night on home visit and then discharge on Wednesday. I am really happy. It is hard to think about anything else really. He was particularly pleased with the way I had recognised the déjà vu moment over the weekend, absorbed it, accepted it for what it was, breathed through it and carried on. He said I did too much on Saturday which I kind of know – it is a reminder of my limitations.

I have a metaphor in my head based on my knee operation a couple of years ago. You go to hospital for the operation and immediate aftercare. Once you are safe after the op you get discharged, but you are not suddenly well again, rather you engage in a long process of rehab and physio to get the knee working. It is weeks before you can run again. Even then, you will still feel it and still need to keep the exercise up to maintain strength – so it is and will be with my head.

There is a funny feeling about being discharged. On the one hand, my progress is great, and it is a good feeling to be going home and getting a bit back to normal. I am so much better than I was two weeks ago. I have not cried in class for several days and have had no major anxiety moments. On the other hand, I will be leaving this safe haven and will have less protection. I will be exposed to the world and that is scary. And it hastens the time when I need to start thinking about the longer-term, which I have kept firmly tucked away while I have been here. I am sure that it is normal to feel in that way but it means the feelings are mixed nonetheless – but I recognise them for what they are, accept and understand them, and move on.

I see now how all-over-the-place my thinking was at that time. I had had a few days when I had managed largely to keep things together while hidden away in a psychiatric hospital. I was going to be allowed out but would still be coming back on a daily basis. It was a very small step on a long road. And yet I was already worrying about when I would need to think about longer-term plans. I still had not realised just how ill I had been, still was, and how long I would need to give myself to get to a point where long-term meant more than the next day.

Tuesday 27th July

So this is the day. I sleep really badly, awake in the dark hours for age after age hoping to be dragged back into sleep before the dawn arrives to greet my still open eyes and, after a few more hours of restlessness, I drag my tired body from the bed to shower and begin the preparation for class. Today I have agreed to meet one of the group for breakfast and then go to town for a coffee. This seems like a big thing to have planned with someone else, the first time I have made a plan to do something with someone that is not just nipping outside for a smoke, or going to the canteen at mealtime.

The morning is psychodrama which is good as always. The issues raised make me think about the positions of me and my brothers, my eldest brother's reaction when the middle one arrived, and his when I came along and took his place on Mum's lap or breast – was this why we fought for so long? And of the positions of my own children. I am also struck by issues around responsibility for someone else's state of mind – that I am not responsible for Lucy's, nor she for mine, nor for trying to make each other better, however much we may love each other, have compassion for each other and empathise.

And so the moment comes to pack and leave. Packing is surprisingly quick – I get a night's supply of meds and am handed back my razor. I pack my bags and scan the room a couple of times for lost socks. I notice a penny left in the desk drawer and decide to leave it as a lucky charm for the next inhabitant. They seem to be coming thick and fast at the moment. Just today there seem to be several new arrivals, some day-patients and some outpatients. I say some goodbyes, but I will be seeing everyone tomorrow, so it is not really goodbye. I sit and have a final chocomilk and fag as an inpatient sitting on the lawn outside. And then I pick up my bag, and wheel my case down the drive.

I am a stark contrast to the shaking, crying, broken man who arrived two and a half weeks ago. Then I was driven to, and gently coaxed through, the door, crawling over the threshold, metaphorically at least. Now I am striding back out into the world, confident of my ability to navigate the rush hour Tube network. It is like leaving boarding school because my parents have returned early or something – term has not ended and I will be back tomorrow but I am getting out and getting home. There is some trepidation – the world is not an easy place and I know Lucy is not in a good place – so it may not be a joyful homecoming, but it is a milestone for me, the end of the beginning of my recovery, a move to the next stage.

Lucy and I sat outside in the evening and drank a bottle of wine and chatted for ages which was lovely. I talked about what I am thinking, and about meditation and all sorts, and she told me how she had been saying all these things to me for ages.

CHAPTER 11

TRANSITION

Wednesday 27th July

It is my first day back as an outpatient at the Priory – a nice feeling, walking in in the morning with a coffee, having time to sit and chat before classes. I got frustrated in the men's support group which seemed to descend into a competition between two members of the group about how much money they had lost and how expensive their previous homes had been. It was a little dull for the rest of us.

More people are moving on. The transience is always there, it can unsettle but it is also a positive reminder that we are all on a journey at different stages. In terms of my journey it feels like maybe the Priory is a station, where we change trains and take a break. I feel like I could get back on the same train – perhaps it is one of the huge night trains that crisscross Europe while everyone sleeps, that stops in the middle of the night at only the largest stations and waits while water and provisions are taken on, and staff are changed. I could get back on the same train again when this time is over, or I could cross the platform and get on a different train going somewhere else at a different pace and for a different purpose.

I am feeling cut off a little from my feelings. I have not cried for some time and when asked how I feel at particular times, I struggle to describe them. It may well be the drugs. I hope it is not me reverting to a state in which I bury or discount them.

Thursday 28th July

My first weekday at home, my first day off. It brings various reminders of how fragile things remain. There is tension with Lucy – me caught between what she wants to do, what I want to do, and what I have been told I should do to look after myself.

Later, having done some phone calls and emails, and phoned my parents and then gone for an hour's gentle bike ride with the dog and kids, I am exhausted and feeling quite vulnerable. It was not a particularly strenuous morning, but it has drained me. I curse the Test and County Cricket Board for scheduling the next test match to start tomorrow and not today (thereby depriving me of a plan for the day) and I take myself off to bed. I cannot sleep, but at least I rest and enjoy some silence away from the noise of kids and others.

In the evening I cook for everyone – it is fajitas so only involved chopping some chicken and veg and frying them with a packet of spices, but I do it nonetheless and it is the first meal I have prepared for weeks it seems. Well done to me.

Later I go out for a beer with my best mate Mike. This is the first time I have arranged a social occasion for two months, the first time out without Lucy for months, and the first time out at all in the evening since becoming an outpatient. It feels like a big event. It is great to see him, and to relax in male, and different, company. During the course of the evening and day I am also reminded of how many other people care – two old friends send texts, two clients get in touch as well as one of my brothers and my parents. I am not alone.

Friday and Saturday 29th and 30th July

We had mixed diagnosis CBT in the morning. This is basically an intro to CBT, working out your own issues and having a first crack at applying the approach which I find interesting. The group is a mix of new and old hands which is helpful. We look at negative automatic thoughts today, challenging negative views or reactions / interpretations to / of events. We break into small groups to analyse each other which I am told I do very well. The more I do of this, the more I wonder whether I could make a career in it. In the afternoon we have assertiveness which for me is all about learning to say what I want – both in the work context and at home, I think. We look at why we have a problem saying no, and techniques to do so comfortably. After the class, which is with my key worker, she asks me for an update, in the midst of which, we talk about a possible career change and she says that she thinks I would make a very good therapist, and that it has come up in conversation between her and others too. Hmm ...

It is the last day for a guy I have become really close to. It is a strange and quite amazing process we have been going through together, looking into the abyss of our hearts, minds, and experience, challenging the very core of who we are, and doing it in front of, and with, each other, nudging each other further forward, guiding each other by the arm when we falter, and reassuring each other at the same time. I am going to places I never knew existed and I am going there with people who were complete strangers a few weeks ago, trusting in them simply because they are here and are doing the same thing.

After hugs goodbye we exchange some cheesy texts telling each other how important we have been to each other on the journey so far and make promises about staying with the journey together – I hope we mean it. After class, a group of us nip to the pub for a pint which is nice – all very normal, no one would know we were on day release from the loony bin. Parents seem quite happy for us to talk to their children, we are given real glasses.

I take the dog for a bike ride and feel tired and anxious. Later in the day (and indeed a bit last night) I am scared. I do not know why, but there is no other word for it. I am shaky and feel like I would be crying were the drugs not numbing my feelings. Lucy is going to France before dawn tomorrow with the kids, so I am going to be on my own. I will have to get to France on my own and have to decide when and how so it may be a combination of all that.

Then there is the work issue – I need to bring them up to date and get approval from the doctor to take another month off. Whatever the cause, if indeed there has to be one, I am jumpy and tense all day.

I try to have a sleep but can't nod off so end up watching some cricket. We do some shopping and I cook a roast chicken which I manage without any real anguish or anxiety, so that is a definite positive for the day.

Lucy's alarm wakes us both at 4.10 and we get everyone in the car, the final bits of packing squashed in, and I wave them off and try for an hour to get back to sleep before giving up and resigning myself to a tired day ahead.

Sunday 31st July and Monday 1st August

With Lucy and the children away, I spend the morning on Sunday with a mix of chores and relaxation. Then I set off to meet my brothers in Oxfordshire for lunch. I have not seen them for weeks and have turned down offers of company down here from them both. I suspect that they are wondering what to expect. We sit outside and have a very nice lunch. It is great to see them. They are calm and we chat and joke in a happy friendly atmosphere. They ask me lots of questions and I feel that it is all about me which is probably not surprising, but I do try to turn the conversation on to them every now and then. Because all I have been doing is therapy stuff, my news and chat is all very much about me, which feels a little selfish, but they are interested and concerned.

When I mention that one of my courses is assertiveness, Pete asks whether that is to be less or more assertive which makes me smile. It is true, I think, that I will assert myself in debate, but not at home and not at work in terms of saying no, or saying what I think or want, because I have no real idea of what it is I do want. I wonder whether some people have really clear and fixed ideas of what they want – I have always assumed they do – but my mind is always filled with thoughts of what other people want and, with no great force of what I want, I go with the former rather than the latter – it avoids having to work out what it is I do want and also any risk of a dispute between the two.

The drive there was manageable. After lunch we went for a walk – there is a hill with red kites around. The suggestion is made

97

that we walk up but I cannot face that amount of exertion and so I persuade them we should drive up and then walk around the top which is relaxing. It takes a bit of effort to convince Pete that I really cannot walk the hill. The energy required just to have got there, to be there, and to resist the temptation to run away as soon as lunch was over, is exhausting enough.

On Monday I have a productive morning – and it's important to pat myself on the back for achievements as well as not to overdo things. I go to the doctor who signs me off for a couple of months. That helps me get my head round being in France for an extended period. It is nice to catch up with the doctor, he is happy to go with what I feel and if, after discussion with the people at the Priory, we feel I may be ready earlier, then of course we can review it. He gives me 28 days of medicine which I realise is not enough if I am going to be in France for a month, but something stops me sorting it out which is daft.

I have a list of other bits and pieces to do which I only manage because of having the list at hand to remind me and then I go and buy a laptop. This is one of those situations where all I know is, I want a laptop. They have tons of them to choose between and somehow, I am going to have to make a choice. They could sell me anything quite frankly, but I hope what I ended up with is alright.

Being on my own is peaceful. I feel in control. It is a bit lonely maybe but that is okay and the peace makes up for it. One of my brothers had wanted to come back with me yesterday so that I would not be on my own, but I find it easier dealing with the world in little chunks, able to turn it off when it's too much.

Tuesday 2nd August

This is my first entry and my first work on my laptop – I have never had one before and this feels very liberating in a funny sense. This is mine, my place, for me to write what I want and no one else has any business with it. I do not need to ask permission to use it, no one can take it away without my blessing nor access what I do on it.

Reading that now seems strange in different ways. First of all, where was I writing my diary before then? I am guessing I must have borrowed a laptop from Lucy, but how did that work? Was I always having to ask to use it? How did I feel able to write so freely when I had it? Secondly, why on earth had I not given myself permission to have one previously, especially since I use it so much now? It is almost as if I had no personal identity. In work I had a computer and was part of the work system. When I came home I was part of the home system. There was no place where I was just me. I know that may seem like it is making a great deal out of an electronic device, but it resonates somehow.

One of the difficult things about the Priory is its very separation from the rest of the world. The conversations you have with people and the relationships you build up are quite unlike anything elsewhere, and in many ways it becomes, or perhaps it has to be, a place that is yours and yours alone, not something to be shared with those around you in the real world. But this can get confusing.

Because the discussions we had with men in there are so different (and I guess because I have never been sexually attracted to men), those interactions felt noticeably different and special. With some of the women, however, the intimacy and understanding, the tenderness and concern you show for each other can easily be mistaken for something else. It's as if your brain tries to reconcile what is happening with past experiences or expectations and says oh, right, yes, I know what this is, this is a relationship developing. No relationship did happen of course – there's the rule book for a start that forbids it – and, more importantly, I was married. There was another factor at play as well though. When I was first ill, Lucy would go with me to many appointments with doctors because I could not go on my own. When there was any discussion of what had led up to my being ill, we talked about the pressures of work, my relationships with people at work, and the various roles I took on outside of work. Once I started having conversations with people on my own, and a lot of time on my own to reflect, my mind began to move beyond thinking solely in terms of issues around my work and extra-curricular duties and to think more about the dynamics of my relationship with Lucy.

In a very real sense, physically as well as emotionally, I withdrew from everything else in my life, the world with which I could cope shrank into myself. I was trying to make sense of things. All of my understanding, certainty, and my confidence about the world and my relationships with, and in it, had shattered. I struggled to make sense of myself and so had no space left to try to make sense of anything else.

Slowly, over the weeks and months that followed, as the fog in my mind occasionally cleared a little, I began to try to make some sense of the wider world. This book is about my illness and recovery; there was a narrative going on alongside that around my relationship with Lucy. The sad truth is that, although we love each other dearly, we are no longer together. Lucy was immense in many ways in supporting and caring for me and as a result she features heavily in the narrative of my recovery. I am trying at the same time to separate out the story of what happened to us – our relationship belongs to us both and is not something for me alone to share.

I think it might be Einstein who said that only a fool keeps doing the same thing, expecting a different outcome each time. My illness shattered every aspect of myself and gave me an opportunity to start again in some ways – indeed I kind of had to. The experience itself and the recovery process changed me, and I knew that I had to change, I wanted to change, if I was to find peace again, if I was to be able to live. And that had to be a personal thing, a process that I did myself.

No one can change you apart from you. It does not mean you have to exclude people, but as you change, the ways in which you interact with others will change. And that creates tension and (I am sure) can be very hard for others (who are used to how you were) to deal with. They did not shape you as you used to be, they are not responsible for how you were or why you got ill, but they will be impacted by your recovery, by the changes you undergo. We are all changing all of the time, of course. Normally it's slow and gradual and two people in a relationship together will quite easily accommodate those little changes in each other as they grow together. A mental breakdown is more seismic than that, I guess, and the rebuilding process that follows can be too much change too quickly for a relationship to survive.

In mindfulness this afternoon I was really quite agitated. A few times while meditating, my hands and arms shook uncontrollably. I was aware of feeling very sad and tearful but not able to cry, which I think is the drugs, and then feeling really anxious and shaking. The guy leading the group suggests that if feelings have been suppressed then it may not be surprising that they come out in meditation and that that is a good sign in that I am giving way to them, which makes some sense.

After class I met a mate for a drink who told me about the mental health struggles his mother had endured – something he had never mentioned before. Another example of what happens when you do start talking about this stuff.

I feel slightly apart from the world. I am not living at the Priory – I come and go from there. At home there is no one else here. I know that I have chosen this, and it is good being able to control what I do and have the peace and quiet and I know that I am choosing something else next week, but nonetheless I am very conscious of the feeling of being in a bubble on my own.

That said, when I got home and the neighbour was having problems starting his car I was able to say to him, and mean it, that although I could not make his car work, if he wanted a lift anywhere then I was happy to oblige – he declined but it felt back to normal a bit – I felt good that I was able to make the offer, and mean it. Small steps.

Wednesday 3rd August
Classes were okay then I went to see the psychiatrist. We talked about how I am feeling a little disconnected generally, feeling that

I am not experiencing my feelings fully, no libido, moments of agitation. He seems okay with my progress. He blames the meds for me not experiencing feelings and the libido issues, and says I have done well to get to where I am.

Saturday 6th August

On Thursday I met Mum and Dad for lunch. It was nice to see them. They were warm and understanding and calm. Mum and I hugged. I shook Dad's hand, but I probably could have hugged him. They have been genuinely concerned about me, I know. We talk about a variety of things, where I go from here, some of the treatment I have been having, the state of the church garden, that being one of Dad's fall-back conversational topics.

We talk about mental illness in Dad's family, his sister and mother in particular. The question of genetics comes up and Dad is quick to confirm that he has never had any problems. I reassure him the issues I have are not linked to the bipolar that seems to have afflicted at least his sister.

I had hoped to meet a friend from the Priory later. It turns out she won't have time. I text her to ask where she will be tomorrow, and she does not reply which sparks an outburst of catastrophising and rumination as I conjure up fears that she thinks I am some leering pervert who has misunderstood friendship for something else and who is trying to impose himself on her, that I have betrayed her and let her down.

It gets to the point that when I am going to the Priory on Friday morning I am fearful that she will have spoken to everyone else and told them what she thinks of me and that I will now be a pariah. When I arrive and there are very few people around, I somehow manage to weave this into the narrative as proof that everyone is hiding away from me.

[My diary goes on in much greater depth regarding this paranoia – I have spared you and me the pain of that!]

In the end, as part of my check-out risk assessment, I do mention this to my key worker who says she is sure there is no problem but that she will keep an eye out.

In the morning in the mixed diagnosis CBT class we had done an exercise in arguing with one's critical self. The theme for the session was reinforcing our positive helpful thoughts – formulating a positive thought to correct something negative (e.g. 'I should not irritate people' gets corrected to 'I would prefer not to irritate people, but I cannot control how people feel, ultimately it is their reaction to a particular event, and in any event I am entitled to look after my own interests as well as those of others.') We then conduct an exercise of arguing this out between our critical and compassionate minds. So, we put out two chairs and switch between the different voices, switching chairs as we do so. It is a little like psychodrama save that it is only ourselves we bring into the room and we do not involve others in role playing. It is amazing how much easier it is to be in the critical chair as opposed to the compassionate chair.

In the course of this exercise a tear or two escape my eyes which I am pleased about. It means I can still feel although I suspect that, but for the drugs, there would have been a lot more tears. I also wonder whether I may be looking at all the learning we are doing at an intellectual level, as an academic exercise, and using that as a shield from applying it too much to myself.

After class we go to the pub. There are 10 or more of us and lots of people say lots of very nice things about me, how I will be missed, the sense I make of things. We part with hugs and exchanges of mobile numbers and promises of staying in contact and thanks and all that. Some of which at least are true! I hope that a number of us do stay in touch. I am taken by how many people are thanking me for my wisdom, candour, kindness, and support.

And so the time comes to leave the Priory. What are my feelings? There is some trepidation. The kind of support and the extent of the support I have there is not available in the outside world, or at least I need to work on my ability to make requests in order to establish it. Perhaps it could be there if I get used to seeking it out. The routine of the Priory is gone for me. I have to fill my time and take my learning forward. I will have no place to run away to, and will be spending a month with the family full-time. I am looking forward immensely to that and to the opportunity for rest, but it is also scary because my needs, and the pace at which I am able to live at the moment, are not the same as theirs, and we will need to learn to marry the two somehow. I need to limit the amount of time I spend on chores each day, set aside time for meditation, exercise, and sleep.

I find myself reflecting on the people I have met and those that I am closest to – I have known very many who have come and gone or been ever-present during my time there. Those I am closest to seem to be based on the normal thing about personality fits but also the happenchance of timing – with whom I overlapped the longest.

CHAPTER 12

REFLECTIONS ON THE PRIORY

The Priory did not cure me. I did not walk out all better. What it did do was stop me getting worse and gave me a safe place to do that. It took away the world so I did not have to worry about it. It also gave me the space, encouragement, and expert support to start thinking about my illness and myself – a process that continues to this day. It gave me tools that I use every day. The sparks lit in me by the Priory led me directly to my own therapy and then through that to study counselling and psychotherapy, to learn more about mental illness and wellbeing and, ultimately, to build my work around it.

It opened my eyes and mind to a whole different way of thinking about and understanding people, how our minds operate, why we do the things we do. It helped me recognise my ability to develop a little self-awareness and to take ownership of how I react to events and to people and, if this does not seem too grand, how to live. If my coach at work had challenged the foundations of all my assumptions to date, I was now beginning to see how those foundations had come about and think about how I might replace them. I realised that this was something only I could do, but also that it was *something I could do.*

In reality I only spent a short time there - less than four weeks in total as an inpatient and then an outpatient. I knew when I was getting to a point when I could and should leave; when I realised those people around me were far sicker than I was, it was time to go. Staying longer than you need will only slow down your recovery.

There are a few words of wisdom from the Priory that I still carry with me. One of the mindfulness therapists would carry a clock with him which he would place on the floor in front of him at the start of each session. It was, in most respects, a normal clock, the kind you would see in many school classrooms. Across the glass covering the face were the letters N, O and W. They made it hard to see the hands and the numbers behind them. He would ask people to tell him the time and invariably people would struggle, unable to see past the letters, and yet unable to see the word and message they spelled out. It was a simple and valuable reminder of the need to spend as much time in the present, not worrying about what has happened or what is yet to come.

Another much quoted favourite was 'This too will pass' - that however painful and hard things seem right now, it will pass. Sometimes it is hard to believe that, but one of the benefits of growing older is that you know the rhythm of things. You do not need to mourn the setting of the sun because you know it will rise again in the morning. Equally, take time to notice and enjoy the good things because they too are transient. Over time that mantra has become a central theme of my approach to life and, as a result, a fitting title for this book.

On one occasion, one of the therapists brought to a group session a great collection of books. We were asked to choose a few that meant something to us. We then whittled the choices down to one book and were asked to pick out a number of words or passages that resonated with us at that time and discuss them with colleagues. Finally, we were required to settle on one word. Mine was "enough". Not in the sense of having had enough of this, but rather the existence of the opportunity or need to give myself permission to say I have tried hard enough, I am doing enough, I am enough – as opposed to constantly doing more and taking on more.

There is a risk of dependency. At various times in the years since, at moments when I have felt most challenged, most anxious, most insecure, when the world terrifies me and I feel unable to cope, I have longed for someone to come along in a van, scoop me up and take me back there. They never have, of course. While I was there, and for a long time afterwards, I wanted to work there, at least part-time, because it felt such a supportive, kind place to be – who would not want to spend time there?

Perhaps surprisingly I have not kept in touch with people from there. Some of us did meet up in the months that followed, but those meetings dwindled and I have not seen anyone for years now. Perhaps the answer is that we all needed to live in our own real worlds again, however changed they might be, and our informal Priory support group somehow undermined that.

CHAPTER 13

ANXIOUS BEGINNINGS

Given that anxiety was to play such a major part of what was to come, it's perhaps no surprise that I have a lot of memories of childhood that are riddled with episodes of fear.

I know I have spent several years in therapy. Therapy is not about trying to blame your parents for everything that has happened. But, in focusing on how you view the world and react to it, and understanding why you have that view and those reactions, inevitably you reflect on early experiences and memories – where many of our patterns of thinking (whether helpful or unhelpful) will have begun. Those patterns of thinking lay down neural pathways in our brains – each time we do something, we create a neural pathway which is there for our unconscious brain to follow the next time we come across the same, or a similar-looking, situation. Subsequently, the years of repetition will have reinforced those cycles of thought, creating new neural pathways for our unconscious to follow.

As a result, you create a narrative of how you came to be who and where you are. By repeating it often enough, that becomes your story, your interpretation of what happened. Born from your own perspective, both then and now, this may vary hugely from that of others at the time (whose recollection now will be coloured by their changed perspective and their own retelling of their narrative).

In exploring my past, therefore, I am doing no more than saying this is my perspective. It is not to accuse or blame anyone. It's just what I thought it was and how I interpreted it. I am also conscious that I am concentrating on the stuff that led me down a path of anxiety, and I would not want anyone to think that was all there was to my childhood.

I am the youngest of three sons. I was born in 1970 and my brothers, Andy and Pete, are three, and four-and-a-half, years older than me respectively. We grew up in Surrey, in a middle-class environment. We had a comfortable (but fairly functional rather than luxurious) house, and a mum and dad who stayed together. Money was tight, but that's because we were educated privately, so a lot of otherwise disposable income went straight to that. We did not starve by any means, but I was conscious that we had a lot less money than most of the other people at school. Holidays in the early years were to Cornwall and then France. The most lavish holiday was a three-week summer trip to Austria, a week of that being spent driving there and back, in the heat wave of 1976, the three of us boys across the red leather back seats of the white Austin 1800 my parents drove at the time.

We were very aware of the sacrifices our parents made for us – Mum worked in order to pay for our education, and they spent little money on themselves. We were also aware of Dad having had a difficult upbringing. It was not that he talked about it a great deal, far from it. What I know mostly came from Mum, I think. Dad's parents had separated when he was still very young, leaving him and his younger sister with their mum who struggled to cope in many ways. From an early age, therefore, he became the responsible male in the house. The money that had supported his education ran out before he could get any qualifications, so he left school and took his exams through evening classes and eventually got himself qualified as an accountant, working for most of his career in-house at an oil company.

Mum had had an easier time of it growing up, and graduated from university in maths. The story has it that someone tapped her on the shoulder and said something along the lines of 'There are going to be these things called computers which are probably going to be quite important, and we need people like you to make them work. Do you fancy it?' And so, Mum became a computer programmer, a job she did for most of her career, bar a short and unhappy phase as a maths teacher.

The Youngest of Three Boys ...

There is a lot of really interesting research and thinking around the importance of where you sit in the family. Middle child syndrome, for example, looks at the dynamics of the middle child who never has the attention and glory the eldest had of being an only child. Then they have their position as the cute baby, getting all the attention and the safety and comfort of the mother's breast / lap, cruelly usurped by the next child to arrive.

As the youngest of three boys, you do, of course, have the benefit of the protective parental arm around the smallest, the most vulnerable. And you never quite lose the ability to seek out Mum's metaphorical lap. You often get the easiest chores to do and your parents have been broken in by the time you arrive and so you may get away with a good deal more than your siblings.

But, you are always available to be a safe punch bag – safe in the sense that you are not going to be able to do any real damage back. You never know as much as them and they can always (probably quite justifiably) decide they have played baby games long enough and are now going to retreat to their grown-up worlds of music, homework, or whatever else.

I still recall something that happened when I was a bit older. Having hit puberty, I was sporting a soft, downy, but nonetheless quite discernible, crop of facial hair. It was time to start shaving. I got some early instructions from my brothers and soon got the hang of it. One day, however, being a good boy who didn't want to cause any trouble, and well aware of the range of punishments available for any misbehaviour, I sought some further advice from one of them. 'You know when you have finished shaving and you have the odd fleck of shaving foam still left on your cheek or neck? Is it okay to wipe that off on the towel, or will it stain it?' I cannot remember the exact response, but it involved howls of laughter and grave warnings of the damage to be caused by shaving foam on towels. I got the message; it was okay.

I also got another message. I felt stupid, humiliated even. From my perspective, I had innocently asked a straightforward question of someone in a better position than me to know the answer, and the outcome was somehow shameful – how could I have been so daft as to think shaving foam might damage towels? So, the message I got was that it's perhaps best not to ask people questions, even those niggling little questions that would take less than a moment to answer, for fear of humiliation. Work it out for yourself and, if you can't, then it is probably better to live with the worry than risk asking a silly question.

I absolutely know that my brother intended no harm to me, that he was just gently teasing me in the way we all do all the time. But I also know this memory is still clear as day in my head more than 30 years later. Looked at another way, it's the difference between intent and impact. The intent was momentary humour while the impact can be seen by the length of that memory. I was made to realise the gulf between my knowledge and theirs.

At school, the moment I told a teacher my name, a glow of recognition (or fear) would ignite their face – oh, another Martin boy. Carving out my own identity meant being different in some way, and for me, that meant working hard and achieving.

But Success Breeds ...

The expectations on you, whether your own or those of your parents, only increase with success. It starts off with a well-intentioned parent wanting a child to fulfil their potential, to do as well as they can, perhaps even to take advantage of opportunities the parent never had. But somewhere along the line it is all too easy for the child to understand that only perfection will do. Being good (because that's what a B-grade was meant to represent) is not good enough; you have to be excellent. In the early days, it is the parents and teachers who impose these expectations, but very soon you learn to do it for yourself – the judging voice becomes your own. And this inevitably breeds anxiety.

Fears of Violence

The early years of private school also held other, more direct, fears. Before that school I had attended a state-funded Catholic primary school. I left aged eight to join my prep school, leaving my classmates to move on in turn to the local state-funded secondary school. I travelled to school by train in those days and our uniform was shorts and a claret blazer – we were pretty easy to pick out, and pick off.

The state school was one more stop down the same train line so that in the morning we would be on the same train, and, after school, they would already be on the train when we were trying to get on. Many of the carriages in those days were made up of a series of separate compartments, each with its own door, but with no way of moving along the train between compartments. So, if you got in a wrong compartment, there was no way of changing until the next stop, and, even then, only if there was no bully preventing you from getting out.

Although the state-school boys had a grudge against all us posh kids, it seemed mine was the greater crime, because I had been a state-school kid who had then gone posh. On enough occasions to cause a fear of repetition every time I got on a train, I would find myself trapped in a single compartment with a bunch of the state-school kids who would threaten, and sometimes act out, beating me up.

Getting home did not mean getting safe. There was the issue of my bigger brothers to worry about – play fighting in the main, but play fighting that rarely ended well for me. There was also Dad.

From the earliest age I can remember, physical punishment was part of the deal. Dad had a pair of leather-soled slippers and, when the occasion was deemed to merit it, the instruction would go out to 'Go upstairs to your room, take your trousers and pants down and wait for me.' After a few minutes he would arrive with one of the slippers and administer a series of hard beatings to my bare cheeks and then leave me to cry it off. It wasn't done in drink and it wasn't generally done in anger, but it was cold and hard, and boy, it hurt. Afterwards there was no element of reconciliation. I was left to cry – perhaps to put myself to bed – and little, if anything, would be said about it again. There was no conversation to bring you back into the fold, to reconcile, or rehabilitate. It was just left there.

Now, I know it was a different age and for many parents and schools at the time this was normal. Also, it was nothing like the violence or abuse that many kids suffer at home. But in terms of what forms you, and informs your perspective, it is what happens to you that is important.

Part of the problem was that there did not seem to be much consistency to it. The same offence might one day result in a beating and one day not. We were generally pretty well-behaved boys, so the beatings were often for offences that were not that serious in the scheme of things – certainly less serious than the stuff you would see your friends getting up to, and some of the stuff we got away with because no one found out.

I cannot now remember how often they would occur, but it was certainly often enough to be a constant threat, an ever-present fear. And the way it was carried out was such total humiliation. It was shaming.

In his book *Healing The Shame That Binds You,* John Bradshaw talks in depth about the nature and impact of shame. He explores the multi-generational effects of how families (dis) function and how children can take on the shame of their parents, preventing their development as complete adults. Because of the shame they feel, they subjugate their own true selves in favour of an assumed identity that will be accepted, and thus lose touch with themselves and grow up to become emotional children in adult bodies. It restricts their ability to form adult relationships and they then create the same effect in their children so that generation after generation are predisposed to the same behaviours. The multi-generational analysis of that in the case of my family is too much for this book, but Bradshaw's book is compelling and well worth a read.

One of Bradshaw's consistent themes is the way in which children feel the need to play a part, to take on roles, to be what they think others want them to be, or what will result in them feeling safe. They thus adopt a personality, a way of being, that is not them. It is not authentic. They become dislocated from themselves. My difficulty with the question, 'But Richard, what do you want?' starts from not really having a sense of self at all – what "I want" is not a question for me, has no meaningful existence for me. It is something to be determined by others and I will then go along with it. When my coach asked me that in early 2011 and looked into my eyes searching for an answer, I cracked, I panicked, because I realised I ought to have an answer and had spent my entire life avoiding it.

Mum went along with the corporal punishment, and would on occasion use Dad's beating herself – 'Go upstairs and wait for your dad to get home and bring his slipper to you.' So, there was no solace or comfort to be had from her and, from what I can remember, the three of us brothers offered no support to each other – when one of us was being beaten, the rest of us would hide away and be glad it was not them.

I do remember clearly how (if not exactly when) the beatings stopped. I was probably about 12. Mum had cooked Spanish omelette for lunch one Saturday when neither of my brothers was around. And I hated it. 'This is disgusting,' I proclaimed after pushing it round my plate for a while and refusing to eat it. I was sent upstairs in a tone of voice that clearly intimated this offence warranted a beating but, instead of being told to wait with buttocks bared, I was instructed to write out 200 times, 'I must not say that Spanish omelette is disgusting.' The age of beating was over – but the messages were mixed because I had always been told to tell the truth, and yet here I was being instructed to confirm, 200 times, my commitment to the exact opposite ...

I am intrigued by the issue of food. I do not have an eating disorder, but I know from speaking to many people who do that it is often used by them as a form of control. When people feel out of control, or don't have a sense of being able to control their own lives, the one thing over which they can exert their control is their food intake. I generally eat well (too well, my weight would tell me). I also eat a fairly wide variety of foods and love cooking. There are a few things, though, which I just cannot eat.

Spanish omelette remains on the dodgy list, but tomatoes are way out in front, closely followed by liver. Tomatoes were loved by both my parents and they grew them in the greenhouse every year. Their taste and texture make me want to gag. I remember having cherry tomatoes pushed into my mouth to try to make me eat them – I refused. Cooked in a sauce they are not a problem, but raw, or cooked whole, I cannot abide them. Liver was something Dad used to delight in. The smell, texture and taste all make me wince and gag. I wonder whether the tomatoes and liver are something to do with early attempts to exercise control in small ways over my diet, in lieu of control over other aspects of life. It may just be my taste buds of course.

The Tongue is Mightier than the Slipper
The physical violence might have ended then, but the verbal violence never really did. There was often a feeling of tension in the air in the house. Dad's way of speaking can often, no doubt

entirely unintentionally, come across as aggressive and violent. 'How much did that heap of rubbish cost you?' was his first response to my brother Pete's first car. He meant it as a joke, I am sure, but the sharp exit of my brother behind a slammed door clearly indicated that was not how it had been taken.

He and Mum seemed to have developed a method of communication which to anyone else appeared designed to wind each other up. I know they loved each other, but it seemed like that love had to be hidden from view.

As the slipper implies, there was a strong sense of authority and discipline. You did not question Dad's view or argue. If you think you are not allowed to express your view or opinion, you suppress it, and in doing so you suppress who you are, because if a little bit of you leaks out, well, people may not like it. Better to say, do, and be, what people seem to like and expect.

As my brothers got older and braver they would confront Dad, and each other, and there would be huge eruptions of anger that would very often result in slammed front doors as someone stormed off and then sudden silence. I would sit in my room not knowing what the argument had been about, or who had been involved necessarily, but just hearing the escalation until the door would bang. And then nothing. No one came to say what had happened or that it would all be okay. There was this very clear rupture with no knowledge about whether it would be healed, or how or when that might happen, but a fear that this time, maybe, things had gone too far and this would be the one that finally destroyed the loose family order that had existed until then.

There was then a distinct fragility to life, a feeling that at any moment things could descend into enormous conflict with unimaginable consequences, and that means that you live with a constant sense of fear. Most of the time you don't notice it because it's what you know, your normal. But every now and then I remember thinking that this felt so contrary to how I somehow thought things should be, that maybe I did not belong, maybe I was not from here, that, despite the physical similarities, maybe I was adopted or fostered. It wasn't that I was hoping for rescue or anything as dramatic as that, but sometimes I did wonder whether at some stage, someone would come along and take me away, back to where I belonged, to where things would make sense.

And Of Course, There is Always God

As a family we went to church every Sunday and I was required to say my prayers every evening. I have had periods in my life when I have been quite religious and felt hugely supported by it … and then there have been other times.

After my breakdown I stopped going to church at all, aside from the odd Christmas visit and funeral. I'm not going to get into a lengthy discussion about my faith but what is relevant is that from very early on, I understood that God sees everything you do, knows what you think, and sits in judgement on us all. If you mess it up, then it's eternal damnation time. That creates a whole other level of fear that even Dad's slipper could not reach – the Heineken of anxiety.

Now, the Catholic Church does allow for confession and forgiveness – but there always seemed to me to be a sense of shame about this – about having to confess your worst deeds and thoughts to a man you couldn't see behind the confessional grille, who spoke to you in whispers. Later we would attend services that involved priests sitting at different places around the church and you would go and make your private confession to them, but in full view of everyone else in the congregation, which just made things worse.

That word "shame" also resonates with the almost ritualised violence of the slipper – waiting semi-naked for the punishment to be administered, without a word and without any reconciliation or pity – if this is what my behaviour demands then I must be truly shameful.

117

Caught Between a Dog and the Old Man with the Rake

Our house was one of three identical houses down a short cul-de-sac, at the end of which were some flats. The road went round those flats in a circle which should have been an ideal circuit for boys on bikes. Also, there was a secret footpath that went from the far end of the flats between the backs of gardens and onto the main road that took you down to the train station, saving a good five minutes compared to walking the long way round on the roads.

The problem was that in one of these flats lived "the old man with the rake". I don't think I ever saw him with his rake. From what I can recall, the flats' gardens were communal and tended by a contractor, so the old man would have had no need for a rake in his flat. I think my brothers were confronted by him (with or without the rake) on one or more occasion. But by the time I was old enough to be exploring my neighbourhood, the legend was firmly established – don't go playing round the flats, or use the secret footpath, or the old man with the rake will come for you.

Years later, I earned some decent pocket money watering the same old man's allotment. He seemed a kindly soul and never once threatened me with a garden implement of any kind – even when he showed me how to use his scythe, I felt quite safe.

At the other end of the road, and guarding the only other exit from our little world, lived a family with two boys, one my age and one slightly older. Years later I would hang out with them, but from when I was young all I can remember about them was the way they controlled my access to and from our street. They had a dog and, whether it was because of the dog being vicious or me being scared of dogs, my fear was that the boys would set the dog on me. Even if the dog was not on patrol, they also had a habit of sitting on their garage roof and catapulting us with pebbles if we dared to try to sneak out of our street.

So, there was fear attached to my little world – I did not live in a constant state of worry about being assaulted by garden implements, dogs, and flying stones, but there was an unconscious sense that the world was dangerous. Added to that was government propaganda at the time which warned of the risks of nuclear war. It seems almost absurd to think about it now, but there really were government information films shown on TV about how to survive in the event of a nuclear strike on Britain. There were threats out there far bigger than dogs and rakes, and worries about them littered my dreams.

There was also the constant threat of Irish terrorist activity.

The threats to our national security today are different but still very real. For my children's generation the iconic image to haunt nightmares might not be a mushroom cloud but rather passenger jets being flown into New York office blocks, or trucks ploughing into crowded streets. I think we perhaps underestimate the effect all of this can have on our individual wellbeing – we think about the anxiety we experience at work and at home, the worries about our health and our finances, our children and friends. But the wider threats from other countries or terrorist groups are almost taken for granted and yet create a constant background music of fear and threat.

Confession Time

I have said that generally we were good kids. There are two incidents, however, when I was naughty – really, properly naughty (okay these things are relative) – and which resulted in such fear that I can still taste it and feel it in every bone of my body.

We learnt the recorder at school. Although almost entirely unmusical, despite being blessed with three very musical children who delight me with their playing far more than they know, the recorder seemed pretty easy. At the risk of insulting recorder players all over, up to grade 5 or so at least, it seemed pretty mechanical and the painful sound you produced still seemed to get approval. So, I did not need to practise that much to get through the lessons. My teacher, Miss Cameron, was an eccentric lady who had long grey hair and smoked a pipe during our lessons. Her two dogs would be part of the class and circle around the assembled boys licking the various cuts and grazes their knees displayed from football and other scrapes.

At some point, Miss Cameron, incensed by the obvious lack of practice from certain members of the class, introduced practice books in which we had to record our daily practice and have it signed by a parent. All went well for a while and I think Mum and I had an understanding that she was not really interested in how long I practised as long as I continued to make progress, so she would readily sign the book whenever requested. I recall the huge trouble other kids got into when they arrived for class without having had their book signed, so it was important to make sure that did not happen to me.

Anyway, on one occasion I was about to go to music class when I realised that I had not had my practice book signed for a week. Then I noticed that my mum's initials were really not that hard to replicate (okay, forge) and so I did what anyone would do (right?) and signed on Mum's behalf. I wasn't really doing anything that wrong because she would have signed if I had asked her to, I'd just forgotten, and the punishment that would have come my way would have been out of all proportion with the offence of being forgetful. And it worked, no questions asked.

But the problem was, once you've started, you can't stop. I knew that if I took my book to Mum to sign for the next week, she would realise that she had not signed the previous week and I would be found out. So, yeah, I started signing for Mum every week from then on and it went on for quite a long time. On one occasion Mum did ask what had happened to the practice books and (in way too deep by this stage to back out) I told her that Miss Cameron had decided they weren't needed any longer and Mum accepted that without question. One benefit of being good is that people do tend to believe you.

All was well until parents' evening came along and I had a sudden image in my head of Mum and Dad going to see Miss Cameron and Mum casually mentioning the demise of the practice book and the whole sorry saga emerging.

Now, this might not, in the great scheme of things, sound that serious, but for me it felt like it might be the end of the world in some way. Whether it was the long-term effect of no longer being trusted, of not being the golden boy, or perhaps a sense that if I could be beaten for what seemed minor transgressions then what the hell kind of punishment would this result in, I don't know. I just could not imagine how this could be overcome, forgiven, and put away so that life could continue. It threatened to rupture absolutely everything. And it was my dirty little secret – there was not another soul who I could talk to in order to gain some perspective.

My experience of parents' evenings up until then was Mum and Dad coming home and saying everyone is very pleased with you, and me then going to bed. This time was very different. All the time they were out I was in a state of complete panic. When I heard their car pull up outside the house I rushed to the front door, desperate to know what had happened.

Trying as hard as I could to be cool, I listened while they went through what the maths teacher had said, and the French teacher, and this and that until ... 'And then we joined the queue to see Miss Cameron ...' My heart was raging, beating a Tube-train-sized tunnel through my ribs. 'It was quite a long queue and we still had not seen your geography teacher ... and it was getting late and we could see that he was free and so we decided not to bother with Miss Cameron and went to see him instead – I hope you don't mind.' The relief I felt, but of course had to hide, was overwhelming.

There is no doubt that I was catastrophising. I suspect it is worse when you are young because you lack control over outcomes and you might not yet have seen what actually happens when you are caught out for something a bit naughty.

With Miss Cameron there was at least a realistic prospect of my being caught, of that conversation between her and Mum taking place in the way I had imagined it. The same cannot be said of my brief foray into shoplifting ...

On the way from school to the train station there were three newsagents, the last of them called Eric Brown. A bunch of my school mates would regularly nick sweets from these shops, which they sometimes shared with the rest of us on the train. Apparently, the trick was to go in with some money and spend some time selecting the sweets you were going to buy, while at the same time stuffing your pockets with whatever else you fancied. Then you went to the counter and paid for what you had in your hand, and smuggled out the hoard that was bulging in your pocket. The purchase was necessary in order to explain why you were in the shop in the first place.

After a long while I was persuaded to give it a go. As I placed my purchases on the counter to be added up by the shopkeeper, a man next to me said, 'And what about the stuff in your pocket, son?' The shopkeeper, while continuing to serve me, asked whether I had anything in my pocket, to which I stammered out, 'No' and was persuaded to pull out my empty pocket to show her. The man then suggested I might like to show the other pocket, at which point I turned scarlet and ran off. No one followed me, perhaps on the basis that my reaction had been enough to assure them that I was never going to be doing that again and had assuredly learnt my lesson.

For months, and I mean months, I managed to convince myself that the shopkeeper would find out who I was, and where I lived, and would write to my parents. Why or how this would happen I have no idea. Much more likely (or perhaps less unlikely) was that she would contact school and I would be identified that way, but somehow the letter to my parents was what I feared. Every morning before school, as soon as I heard the post being delivered (it seemed to come earlier in those days), I would rush to the front door to see if there was something that might have been from Eric Brown. How I was supposed to tell the source of the letter from the envelope I am not sure. Equally, I have no idea what I would have done had there been an envelope that identified itself as the one. What I am sure about is the terror that filled me every morning that this might be the day when the letter arrived, and everything changed forever.

(There is at the back of my head a very small but still lingering worry that Eric Brown might read that and write to my dad – I will risk it!)

Solace in Success at School

I have said that I did well at school. That seemed to keep me safe at home. It meant that I was welcomed and liked by teachers and, as I got older, could develop safe and interesting relationships with them. I was ever conscious of the sacrifices my parents had made to pay for my education so there was a sense of repaying them for that. There was also a growing sense in which achieving academic success would give me a way out. I wanted to escape from where I was. I wanted to get away from home and from school, and academic success seemed to be the best way to achieve that.

And so it proved. I left school with a sack of prizes and A-grades and secured a place at Cambridge to study law. I am not entirely sure why I settled on law. I do know that by the age of 16 that was the plan because it came up in my O-Level Spanish oral exam – I said it was because I liked arguing, but that probably spoke more about the limitations of my Spanish than anything else. I think I had a sense of wanting to be part of a profession. Accountancy was out because my dad did that, medicine needed biology, which I had given up aged 14, or chemistry which I struggled with, so law seemed the right thing. There was also something around service, helping people, resolving conflict, and also about justice, standing up for the little man (against his older brothers perhaps)!

Twenty Years Later ...

Like many professions and careers, law firms have this uncanny ability to keep you forever unsatisfied, striving for something just out of reach. You start off as a trainee and your goal is to qualify as a solicitor, because that is, after all, what you have been progressing towards these last several years of study. So, you work hard to get through that barrier. But when you do, rather than being able to rest up and take comfort in having climbed this peak, you realise that this summit was an illusion. You really haven't got very far at all, and right in front of you is this much bigger mountain to climb called partnership.

It is slowly changing in some firms at least, but when I was coming through there was an expectation that your career had to be always progressing – it was up or out – and so you had to shoulder your backpack once more and climb the partner mountain, or leave. If you don't have the courage or imagination to think about an escape route, there really isn't a choice. But it's okay, you think, because once I have climbed that mountain, I really have made it, I've done it and I can relax a bit.

But it's not like that at all – you haul yourself up those last metres and turn the corner expecting to be able, finally, to sit down and rest at the partners' dining table (metaphorical or real) and then you see that it's still not the end – the range of peaks continues, getting ever higher, stretching far into the distance.

As I say, that's probably true of many careers and organisation structures but the effect is to keep you on your toes, keep you driven, keep you anxious at all times. And because most law firms operate very much on an annual cycle, your position is only as safe as your most recent financial performance. You end one financial year and face the music in terms of how you are deemed to have performed, and immediately you are in to the next year, albeit your performance figures have been reset to zero and you have to prove and justify yourself all over again, only this year with higher targets.

And while you are climbing the mountains at work, you are building a life on the back of them. You work in London so unless you want to have a horribly long commute to add to the hours you already spend in the office, you need to live somewhere within an hour or so of the office, in an area that feels safe for you and your growing family. That costs a lot of money. So, you end up with a chunky mortgage to pay for the house. That's okay because your income is increasing. And then, although the local state primary schools are good, the secondary ones around you in London are not, so (in our case at least) you decide to send your kids to private secondary school.

So now, in order to maintain your life – the school fees, the mortgage, and everything you come to expect for working so hard – you have to earn a huge wad of cash, which means staying in your job – unless you can see (which inevitably you can't) some way to break the vicious circle.

This was never, ever, how I expected or intended my life to be. I am not saying it is wrong. It's just not how I planned it – partly because I didn't really plan it; I did what was expected, I played the role, but if I had any dreams of what my life as a father, husband and lawyer was like, it wasn't that.

There is also something about the nature of legal practice which I think is worth exploring. At the Priory, we discussed negative automatic thoughts and many of those are fundamental to the way lawyers work. The reason for example, why a lawyer will turn a simple agreement to buy or sell a house or a company into a lengthy sale and purchase agreement is because of the need to cover every possible eventuality, to deal with every risk – to catastrophise in other words. Lawyers may well practice as part of a firm, and perhaps within a team within a firm. There are collective responsibilities, but lawyers also have a very strong sense of their personal obligations to the client, to the profession, and to the Court system. If I act unprofessionally, it is my neck on the block as well as that of my firm. This can easily develop into personalisation.

Lawyers generally act for one party against another, and will argue their client's case accordingly, in a manner that can often be black and white in nature. Perfectionism is a recognisable and diagnosable disorder. It can often seem de rigueur in a law firm.

Also, the issues with which lawyers get involved for their clients will almost always have strong emotional aspects to them. Lawyers operate in highly charged environments and yet have to appear dispassionate, professional. That can take its toll, especially when you become more senior and have less opportunity to chat things through, discharge whatever you are carrying emotionally, with a senior colleague.

None of this is to criticise lawyers – they are just some of the characteristics, and risks, of the trade. And lawyers will not be alone in that. Like other professionals, lawyers are trained to put their clients' interests ahead of their own. When someone asks for help we jump to it. We help other people before we worry about ourselves. If we are successful, we have lots of people to help, and less and less time to look out for ourselves.

Learnt Behaviours

Once you have developed a way of being, especially one that seems to have served you fairly well, you stick to it. Your adult relationships, your ways of being with people, reflect those you learnt as you developed. I have had bosses who, I now realise, I treated like my dad. They may not have carried the threat of physical violence, but I feared them in the same way. In the heat of an argument Lucy would shout at me, 'I am not your dad' because the look on my face was clearly one of fear that she was going to beat me. And I go along with what people want because that's what I have learnt. One of the questions that comes up again and again in my therapy is where my anger is. It is incredibly hard for me to access my anger because it is associated so very closely with fear. For me the two are synonymous. I am terrified of my anger because to show it will result in punishment. To show it means to show myself, and I learnt to keep that hidden.

In a conversation between my senior partner and Lucy while I was at my worst, he reflected on how I had always seemed so keen to take on roles and jobs – that whenever something needed doing, I was putting myself forward to do it. When Lucy reported that back to me, I was amazed – my experience had been completely different – that I was being asked to do all those roles. The reality, I suspect, is that when people talked to me about the requirement for things to be done, my desire to please, to be helpful, to be good, as well as my going along with what others wanted, meant that I understood it to be a request for me to help, which I therefore did.

CHAPTER 14

ESCAPE TO THE CAMPAGNE

I had left the Priory, and I was learning to take each day as it comes. I was no longer trying to plan ahead, and I certainly wasn't making any assumptions about how I was going to feel from one sundown to the next. There was certainly a great deal of uncertainty about my leaving hospital, and then England, on the train to the house in France.

I am in a bit of a state about getting ready to go away. I think it is the general agitation and nervousness about leaving the Priory and going to France. I am also sleeping very badly at the moment, which does not help.

I was particularly bad this morning. I woke before dawn and never really got back to sleep. This was after having gone to bed shortly before midnight, despite all my better plans and intentions. I found myself checking locks and windows and all sorts, before I could go to bed and, when I did go upstairs and got undressed, the button came off my shorts and I decided that I had to sew that on again before I could try to sleep. I have been very shaky and nervous this morning.

The journey itself felt like a huge challenge, manageable only if broken down into little chunks – beginning with getting packed and double checking I had what I needed. Then there was the walk to the station, followed by a train to Vauxhall. Next, a Tube train to King's Cross St Pancras. Then navigating the customs and other processes to board the Eurostar. Then the train to Paris. A Tube journey across Paris and then a train from Montparnasse to Angoulême, the nearest TGV stop to our home in the Charente. If I thought about the entire journey, or even all of those individual steps, it seemed impossible, way beyond me. Only by taking one piece at a time could I imagine being able to cope – although there was in the back of my mind the sense of joy and relief I hoped to feel when I arrived at Angoulême and collapsed into the embrace of my family.

That embrace, however, had its own fears. I was straight out of the calm and safety of hospital and living quietly alone at home. I could control everything – nothing need happen without my feeling safe about it. For example, if I needed complete silence then I could have it. I could not expect that same level of calmness and control with the rest of the family, and indeed this was precisely the point – I needed to see if I could start to reconnect with the rest of my world. I had to do this, however hard it seemed. And part of me was thinking you need to start showing your kids that you are still there, that you can be you, and they can have you, and depend on you.

So, chunk by chunk, I made my way. After each stage, I gave myself a moment to stop, take stock, give myself a bit of a pat on the back for the achievement, and then focus on the next stage, get clear in my head what I needed to do and how I was to do it, then a deep breath, and off we go. And it worked. I made it.

The other big fear was that we had house guests – a family that I knew very well and love dearly, but even so, they would be there, when I arrived and for the first days of my time there. I would have to deal with the noise, the rhythms of other people, the challenge of finding solitude and the fear of my need for it being perceived as rude. I would need to be a host somehow, looking after other people when I was barely (if at all) able to look after myself, and always there was the fear of being overwhelmed – of ending up sitting down some place and just crying and shaking.

Was this really just a crazy idea? But it felt like so much depended upon it – it was the first step away from being in an institution, a step that had to be taken at some stage and I knew that it was time to do this, however terrifying it seemed.

Monday 8th August

Shit shit shit shit shit! Have been in France for two days now and the seizures have started again. I have not had one properly since first going to see the psychiatrist at the beginning of June. Today I have had three or four over the last few hours since lunch – it is now half past four. I had one and took myself off to bed where I lay unable to sleep and had a series of them. Familiar faces, voices, phrases. The feeling of weakness and a feeling of intense heat inside of me like I was boiling. I have not noticed this sensation before.

It feels like my mind is a telephone exchange in which all of the wires have been connected wrongly, the conversations all confused. Connections are being made between events, memories, feelings that have no relation with each other. Someone says something which reminds me of some image, which in turn reminds me of some feelings, which have no relation to either. Memories or images that I have seen or felt or dreamt recently being jammed up against, juxtaposed, almost crushed together, with other feelings and thoughts to create a maddening, insane, and senseless jumble of confusion and blur.

I also have big memory problems. I cannot remember what day it is, what happened when, who said what, what is happening to whom and when.

I have been acting a bit like I am better I suppose. I arrived on Saturday and was up until 1.00am chatting, drinking, and smoking. Last night was not as late but was probably still nearly midnight. I wake early in the morning and do not really sleep after that.

I have been doing mindfulness exercises. Three exercises yesterday totalling around half an hour and a 25-minute meditation today without any guidance, just me.

The images and voices feel like they are from the last few weeks. They seem recent and dreamlike, they are not about the Priory but they seem somehow imbued with learning or sensations or references from there – so are they dreams I have been having while there? I feel like the Priory is a long way away. I feel very alone. I was unsure whether to tell Lucy, although I have – it was impossible to hide it. But why did I not want to tell her – because she will worry, blame herself, make herself unhappy? Maybe it is all those things and more, perhaps also because I felt so unhappy about it myself, angry and also worried?

I feel very confused. My sense of place, of time and days, of events that have happened, of what is going on around me, is confused, disorientated. I also feel debilitated, not able to function as I should. I have feelings of guilt, of the passing of time unfilled with activity. Then contrary thoughts about how I must rest, then thoughts about the need to join in, be part of what is happening.

This is a bad place I am in and the fact that it is happening here in France again does not make it any better ...

Wednesday 10th August (Morning)

Yesterday was a black, black day. The visions, the seizures, were with me all day. At times it felt that they were ever-present, no gap between them. The children, the dog, all sparked off memories or visions. The dog reminded me of someone I have seen in my visions that had a face like hers – that could have been a dream. The kids in particular would say things or do things that brought up very distinct memories of events, conversations, times in hospital where they could not possibly have been, or known about, so how could they bring them to mind? It is torture. I feel I am being driven mad by it. And it is all the more upsetting that it is the things, the people, I love that are causing it.

I am clinging to the hope that it is tiredness and / or excess of alcohol that is doing it and that, with our guests gone, I will be able to develop a more controllable cycle of life. I am told that I am doing too much. I need to go off for time on my own which is not just meditation time, but simply peace, away from the questions, the squabbles, the requests, and the noise.

My mind drifts to living here and having animals and then worrying about whether foxes would eat sheep, and how to protect the hens, and how to flatten the land. Jobs, jobs, jobs, worries, worries, worries, thoughts, thoughts, thoughts, plans, plans, plans, and they all drive me to distraction, to madness.

I walk the dog. She hunts out rabbits and hares that she chases across my path. I think of having a gun to shoot them and then think no, it would be too easy in a moment of mental torture, to turn it on myself. The temptation would be too strong. I think about the woods I am walking through, and hanging myself from a tree, and the thought of the children being sent to look for me because I have been away too long – and them finding me ... But then I think Lucy would not send them, she would come herself so that's okay – except, of course, that is not okay.

I feel I may know how my colleague from hospital who died may have felt, or at least I understand it. Here I am, having been through the programme at the Priory, and I am as bad as ever, having seemingly gone miles backwards in the few days since I have left there. I cling to the things I learnt there – breathing, meditation, mindfulness, in the hope they will give me strength, or at least peace. Meditation too easily, however, provides a place for the visions to come back to haunt me, so one of my sessions yesterday was interspersed throughout by the blackness.

I have been thinking about Lucy and how it would be completely reasonable for her to leave me. She does not have to put up with this and, although I cannot imagine being without her, I would understand if she left me and so I tell her. She reassures me she has no plans, although we have talked this morning about the possibility of me going back to England. She talks about the pain of seeing me like this, for her and for the children, of having to keep telling me not to do things, and the frustration at me saying I can do something, and then ending up in a seizure, in blackness.

I go to bed at 10 or so I think, leaving Lucy up. It feels like I toss and turn all night. Eventually, at seven, I give up and get up. I breathe in the morning sun, meditate for half an hour, wash up from last night, get breakfast out, read my book for an hour, and at half-nine the rest of the family starts waking and we start the day together. It is now 11.15 and I have not had any blackness yet ...

I am conscious of how causally it seems that suicide is thrown in to the middle of that diary entry. I guess that reflects how normal a thing it was for me to think about. As I have said, it is very much part of the conversation you have with health professionals on a regular basis and so also becomes part of your own self-checking. But more than that, the overwhelming pain, the abject misery, the complete erosion of all feelings of being safe, or able to cope and continue that I was feeling meant that suicide was absolutely an obvious solution. I cannot bear living and therefore I need to die. The only remaining thought is then about how will it be for those you leave behind – which I guess is what saves you in the end. I could not bear the thought of my children finding me dead, or knowing that I had died, because of what I thought that would do to them. Which means they saved me, albeit unknowingly. It is not that I lacked a purpose for living, I just did not think I was able to do it, to bear the pain of it. And that pain, despite not being physical, is so very real, so completely destructive.

But those thoughts are a current reaction to a current perception of a current state of affairs. All will change – this too will pass. Thoughts are just that – thoughts. They do not have to be acted upon. They will change.

Slowly we learnt to live around each other once more, carefully. On one occasion, we were off with another family to have lunch somewhere, and halfway down the drive Lucy could see that I was not coping and suggested I stay behind which I was relieved to do. When some other people came to visit I had to stay a bit separate from them, half listening to the conversation but half in my own world.

I feel people being unsure around me, not sure what to make of me and uncertain how I will react. The children and Lucy are certainly on their guard, worried lest anything they do should set off a reaction in me, and I do not blame them.

Today they have gone off to meet friends who are camping nearby. They were supposed to visit us here, but Lucy decided that I was not up to it. I am grateful. This is a haven and the fewer people that disturb it the better.

It is very hot. The sun is bright and high in the sky. The sky is blue with a few wispy clouds that burn away by the afternoon. The light is sharp, making the outlines of trees very focused. There is a gentle breeze. I can hear the occasional crowing of a cockerel, the odd bleat of sheep and sometimes a distant mooing from a cow. Somewhere someone is running a tractor. Every now and then a light aircraft buzzes across the sky. Otherwise it is quiet save for the rustling in the huge tress we have around the house that provide us and it with shade from the sun's heat.

There is work to be done. Some things need fixing. A field needs mowing. The animal pens need strimming. But none of this is vital and if it does not get done this week, or next, or at all, it will be okay – no one is in any danger.

I have had no seizures for two whole days now and that is an enormous relief. I continue to be haunted by the prospect of them returning, the memory of their agony, my head and my whole body being torn up and burnt by them. But for now, they are away. I was anxious this morning, caused by the (short) list of things that needed to be done while everyone was away. I also started the day with a trip to town rather than a meditation. I managed the trip and finally meditated in the bright sun for half an hour without any commentary, just me, focusing first on my breathing, then my thoughts, then the sounds around me, then my body and what was supporting it, and the pressure points between my body and the sunbed I was lying on. I returned to my breath and for the last few minutes felt at peace, calm, in a true state of openness, awareness, and acceptance. I could notice thoughts as they came and passed across my mind without any effort on my part, and then nothing. Then a sound that came and went, or another thought passing across, and then nothing – and so on. Afterwards I felt re-energised and able to tackle the things that needed doing.

After some awful nights where I seemed to sleep for only short periods, if at all, Lucy asked if we could sleep separately. She needed the space to be on her own, not worrying about me and noticing my lack of sleep or agitation. She said I had been shaking in bed as well as having funny breathing and leg twitching. I was reluctant at first because I need her and do not want to create barriers between us, but I agreed for her sake and, in fact, we both sleep much better like this. The last two nights I have slept right through I think and not woken until eight or even later so that is much better, although I do not know how long these arrangements will last. I do not want them to be permanent.

I exist here. I eat and drink and sleep. I can interact with the family and take myself away. I have to do nothing and that is good. England, work, the Priory, all seem a very long way away and the thought of returning to any of them is distressing. I miss the Priory though, the people, the gentleness, the safety, the talk, the routine. That and the people there were all I was for several weeks, and now they are all gone from me and I feel an emptiness as a result.

Without trying to plan or think about things or worry, I seem to have come to an awareness that I may not be able to go back to work. That life, that person I was there, seem alien to me. I do not know who or what I am now though. A visitor from England and I were chatting, and he said he was in HR and I found myself saying I am an employment lawyer, but at the same time thinking maybe I used to be an employment lawyer. I certainly am not the person I was when I was last there and that seems such a long time ago.

To think that I have not been there since May and all the things that have happened to me since then … it seems a huge void, an unbridgeable chasm. I do not know if that is fear of going back or simply a moving on. I am being changed by all this, but a new person has not yet emerged. We were talking to the kids yesterday about the metamorphosis that caterpillars undergo to become butterflies in the chrysalis and perhaps that is what is happening to me. I am cocooned, having built my chrysalis from all that has happened and at some stage I will emerge. But not yet.

Sunday 14th August (Lunchtime)
The day starts dreary and rain soon arrives. It seems to reflect my mood. I woke anxious and remain so still. Meditation did not seem to help. I went to the supermarket with Steph and coped but was ill at ease. Some England friends' kids are here. Later, another family from England will arrive and we will be entertaining 17, including ourselves. Ambitious with the sun shining, but more so in the rain. There will be little respite from the noise and bustle and stress of other people. With the rain I cannot even walk the dog as an excuse to get away from it all.

Yesterday I took the kids to the lake beach at Brossac and left Lucy at home. The kids swam then we played crazy golf and had lunch, a bit of reading and then home again. I guess we were out for six hours which was a good break for Lucy. The day before, I strimmed the animal pens. I am not entirely sure why – we do not have animals to keep in them. I think it is a combination of things. It makes the place look tidy, it feeds the dream that one day we might have animals, but most of all it allows me to feel I have some control over things, and can keep my own land, without always having to rely on other people to come and do things.

I was struck by the atmosphere in the local auto horticulture shop. It is a big place with tractors, ride-on mowers, power tools and all sorts. It is staffed by a never-ending run of burly French men of a certain age, many sporting moustaches, who all look like they can fix anything, would know just the right tool for any kind of job and would have used them all in their time.

Other French men come in with things that need fixing, twisted bits of metal or whatever. There is a general greeting to all and sundry with big handshakes to the staff as if they are long lost brothers. It seems more like a community centre than a shop.

As I write I am sitting inside but next to a floor-to-ceiling window, wide open looking out onto our barn with a door painted the traditional pale blue / green of the Charente. The wall is a slightly crumbling stone and mortar affair, the stones a seemingly random assortment of shapes and sizes. The only regular shapes surround the door. A hydrangea is in flower in front of my window and there are various herbs and flowering shrubs in a bed by the barn. The dog hops in and out of the window. A fly is buzzing around my head, birds are nattering to each other in the fruit trees, there is an occasional splash and scream from the kids in the pool on the other side of the house and Lucy has just brought me a cup of coffee. Despite the gentle drizzle it is hard to imagine a more peaceful scene. My spirits rise a little as I take it all in.

It is hard to know what causes my mood to rise and fall. Yesterday had been a good day all told, little anxiety and another day free from the darkness of the seizures. I went to bed relatively early leaving Lucy, Steph, and Gina watching TV. I read for a while in bed before turning in. I did wake a few times in the night but had a fairly decent sleep and woke for the last time around eight or so. I am feeling some anxiety around more people coming to stay.

It is just a little scary, the fear of being overwhelmed, of being overrun by the noise and bustle and the need to talk to them and do things at their pace. I have not seen them since I was ill. The parents will be very concerned, and probably quite gentle, so there is no reason to fear them, and if I need to disappear for a period they will understand and cover for me. I suppose the reality is that until coming here we have not had people to lunch / dinner / stay, or any combination of those, since May. I have been wrapped in cotton wool in my own little cocoon with the rest of the world kept at a distance, and now it is encroaching on me.

Wednesday 17th August (Late Afternoon)

Today has been unbearably hot and the forecast is for it to get hotter.

Like yesterday, I began the day with half an hour of meditation.

It was hard to keep a focus and stop my mind from going all over the place. But I have learnt to accept that as part and parcel of it and not a failure. It does not mean that the time has not been well spent. I am rarely achieving any higher state of insight or peace, but the time itself is peaceful and calming and leaves me more able to face the day.

I followed up with a run. The dog came with me and then lay on the cold tiles of the kitchen floor afterwards to cool down. Running makes me feel more like my old self, more in control of my body, more manly in a funny sense.

This morning continued busy as I went to get the chainsaw fixed, buy food, petrol, a kettle, a Hoover, and some other bits and pieces. Although I was tired this afternoon and did some sitting around, I do not feel too bad and am pleased that I seem to be able to add a little more activity. Our house guests have been and gone and tonight an English couple from down the road are coming to dinner.

A huge oak tree shed a massive branch in a storm the other night – the reason for getting the chainsaw fixed. Once the wood is chopped we will have enough for the winter and a few more after that, I reckon.

I still find home, work, the Priory and England a million miles away.

Would it be a terrible and unforgiveable waste of a brain and an education to spend my life doing manual work around here? Who would judge me, and am I answerable to them? Can I simply make the decision? Do I need permission? And what is the decision – it might be simply to stay here for a bit and see what happens. What about the psychotherapy that was exciting me a few weeks ago?

I have picked some of our pears today to make a tart to follow on from a butterflied leg of lamb marinated in our own rosemary (among other things). We have lovely figs that are ripening now and peaches still to come. There are numerous different sorts of apple, a quince tree, and wild blackberries – we are self-sufficient in fruit. We could easily keep hens for eggs and livestock for meat and other needs. It would be such a change and such fun. But have we, have I, got the bravery for it?

Sunday 21ᵗʰ August (Morning)

Just back from a run again, before which I meditated for 20 minutes looking into the dawn. I am sitting outside the front door on the gravel terrace. The air is cool, the sun still behind clouds and low in the sky, and there is a definite breeze. Yesterday the heat was intense, stifling. We ended the day skinny dipping in the pool (just Lucy and me) while the kids watched TV after supper. I guess that says something about my state of relaxation that I was willing to do that – that is not the stressed, preoccupied, anal and obsessed Richard Martin that we are used to. Lucy says that my face is much more relaxed, it is not grey, my eyes are more alive, the frown lines gone – and I have a tan which always helps.

All that heat yesterday was followed by a storm in the night. The wind got up and then the rain came down. This morning there are various branches broken from trees (but all small ones, mercifully) and our temporary ground coverings made up of AstroTurf and the old pool cover have been re-arranged. Otherwise there is no apparent damage, but it does remind me of the realities of living in the country – real things happen here.

As I write, a cockerel is bidding me good morning from the neighbouring farm (yes, yes, I heard you the first time and good morning to you too), a pigeon is cooing and there are various birds in the lime tree above my head tweeting merrily to each other. The dog is lying at my feet under the table, recovering from the run. Every now and then her ears prick up at the sound of a lizard scuttling through the leaf debris or up the wall of the house. Everyone else is still in bed, asleep as far as I can make out. I saw no one on my run – this morning belongs to me.

Jude has woken up – I can hear him singing Daniel Powter's 'Bad Day'.

Mentally I have been fairly good over the last few days with the one exception of Thursday where I had a couple of seizure episodes. I think the fact of the volume of wine and lateness of bed the night before with the neighbours (I do not, of course, mean bed with the

139

neighbours, more that they kept us from our bed) has probably got
a lot to do with it and there have been no recurrences since. I have
had a few moments of mild anxiety and quite a lot of just feeling
depressed, low, numb.

I am also still not sleeping well. Last night I was in with Lucy after
a few nights sleeping separately, but in neither place am I sleeping
for more than an hour or two at a time. Last night was particularly
bad – it took ages to get to sleep, first because of the heat, meaning
I was dripping with sweat, and then the wind and rain. Even after
the storm, I was awake for a long time and woke every hour or so
through the rest of the night.

I am reading a lot, and able to concentrate for a good while
reading. I am also able to see through a game of Scrabble which is
not something I could do a few weeks ago.

There is progress in these entries, but nothing linear. Sleep
might improve for a few days, then get worse again, but overall
the change was positive. I was able to relax and I was also able
to engage with people and with tasks, set goals and achieve
them. My love for the place was deepening all the while. It felt
like the only place on earth where I was safe, where I could
possibly want to be, the only place where I could be. I felt like I
was becoming part of it and wanted to look after it as it looked
after me. I was also learning just to be.

At the same time, reading this now I see the things I was not
aware of, the bits I had missed while I checked out or checked
in at the Priory. The swimming pool had been replaced. But, of
course, that was not because the old one had decided to move
on and a new one happened to be passing by and nestled itself
in. Lucy had organised it. I vaguely recall her asking me about
it at times earlier in the summer, but I could not engage and
left her to it. She got on and organised it.

That English couple from down the road sound in my entry
like new people we had just met. In fact, he (a mechanic and
part-time builder) had been passing by one day while the new
pool was being installed and had intervened to point out that

without a retaining wall, once the new pool was filled there would be nothing to stop it sliding down the hill, and so had got in touch with Lucy and they had agreed he would build the required wall. When Lucy and the kids arrived, they had filled the pool and then worried about the state of the pool surround and whether that would upset me. So they had bought up every piece of AstroTurf within 20km of the house to cover the bare earth and rubble. I had been absent for all of this.

The other day something made me check the Google Earth view of the house. For years it had been an old image, the old pool still there years after it had been replaced. Now a new image is there, the new pool, the football goal I built on what we now call the football pitch, the trampoline we brought over from England, and in the bottom field I am mowing.

CHAPTER 15

THE END OF SUMMER

Friday 25th August

It has been a few days since I last wrote anything and therein lies a tale. I am writing sitting in our covered outdoor eating area at the back of the house, looking out over our fields. I did a load of mowing yesterday, including the field I can see. I have also been busy decorating inside the house and doing various manual labours outside.

I can also see our washing dancing jauntily in the breeze on the washing line. My view is slightly obscured by the peach tree that grew from a stone discarded by Madame some years ago.

We have had rain the last couple of nights. There were big storms with thunder and lightning. The lightning helped me lock up last night in the dark as it flashed on to show me the doors and locks that needed closing. We could see the storm miles off and watched as it approached and then circled our house and village. It rained all morning, but we went to a market and brought home hot roasted chicken which we had in sandwiches for lunch with crunchy lettuce and mayonnaise in crusty paysanne bread. We also bought cakes for pudding. Later we will have mussels for supper. Jude is so keen on them that he wanted to spend his own money to buy them. The girls bought yet more bracelets.

I have been keeping up with my meditation. My mood has been good – I have felt able to take on all sorts of things – the jobs, phoning people, speaking French. There was one call I needed to make which seemed a turning point. It was not a scary call but one I would have asked Lucy to make, due to anxiety, until a few days ago. I was on the point of asking her to do it and thought no, I can do this, and went ahead and did it. She has noticed the change in me too. I feel empowered, enabled, strong, both physically and mentally. A few days ago, I played Scrabble again with Lucy, was roundly thrashed, but was pleased to have been able to play. Yesterday we played again, and I beat her and notched up two seven letter words and over 400 points.

Today, however, is a different matter. This time next week we will be on our way home and that is a dreadful thought. I feel so free, so relaxed and calm here. The thought of London and all that awaits me there is terrifying. Lucy casually mentioned, as we drove off this morning to market, that this time next week we would be homeward bound, and I have felt very unsettled ever since, particularly after we got back here, and the house threw its welcoming, warm, and promising embrace around me. I belong here and the thought of being elsewhere is grim.

Wednesday 30th August (Late Afternoon)

It has been a good few days since I last wrote. There has been a certain mania of activity.

I took the kids quad biking at Guizengeard which was fantastic fun. After a slow circuit with the instructor and the kids, I was left to play on a proper dirt track with jumps and all sorts. It was so exhilarating. Hours afterwards I was still smiling as the adrenaline left my system.

(Guizengeard sounds like somewhere from Tolkien's Middle Earth, a place where you will find your destiny and good will finally triumph over evil. Except that in French it is pronounced more like geese on guard, and is a fairly barren abandoned quarry which has been made into a lake.)

I have cleaned the house with the kids. We washed all the bedding and hung it out to dry. It is so hot that with a gentle breeze it takes half an hour for washing to dry here. We have had paving slabs for the pool area delivered – and each had to be taken off the delivery van by hand. They are not going to be laid until next year but were on offer in the shop. Unloading it was agonisingly hard work and there is a further instalment on its way. I reckon it must be a ton and a half already with the same to come. I am having second thoughts now about my enthusiasm for helping lay them in due course.

(That last sentence tells a tale. I was a lawyer who worked in the city. Yes I liked a bit of DIY, but anything remotely tricky or big and I was handing it over to the professionals, and people who have real muscles. Here I was saying I wanted to get involved in helping lay the paving stones. When the time actually came to lay them the following year, I just went ahead and did it on my own. My view of who I was and what I could do had changed markedly.)

Saturday and Sunday involved lots of activity outside. On Monday I lit the bonfire which burnt for hours and smouldered for many more, despite the water I poured on it to put it out. I cleared the remains and flattened and raked the ground, preparing it for grass seeding when the rains come, and then mowed the entire bottom field, the front lawn, and the perimeter path (the last bit was in fact done by Jude, with me jogging along behind to make sure he did not get into any difficulty). All that is left are the few pasture areas we have decided to leave for wild flowers, perhaps to be mown by a local farmer for hay before the winter comes.

I feel that in some ways I am becoming master of this house and its land. We are beginning to shape it to our own design. And with each step I fall more in love with the place. From talking to local people, we gather that Monsieur Violel had lots of offers for the house before we bought, many at higher prices. He turned them all down until we came along. We like to think he was waiting for us, that the house was waiting for us, for the right buyers to come along, people who would love the house as he did. Which we do.

Amidst all this activity how have I been feeling in myself? I clearly have a lot of energy back and am enjoying the challenge of things to do and the satisfaction of jobs completed. I guess my feeling of mastery over the house also has an element of feeling more in control of myself and more empowered – stronger, more able. I felt quite anxious the day of the bonfire. I put this down to a mixture of the hard work the days before, shifting over 20 wheelbarrow loads of earth to finish moving the mound, and the slight stress of the fire, anxious to keep it under control. Otherwise I have generally been okay.

Thoughts of going home are deeply depressing. I feel so happy, calm, and at home here and the thought of our London home, or worse still, the office, is scary and feels unnatural – why, when I am so happy here, would I want to go somewhere else – for who or for what would I be doing it? There is happiness here that simply does not exist elsewhere.

I am drinking too much – a bottle of wine each evening plus a beer or a Pineau or two which is not clever, but it is what we do – we sit around outside chatting, drinking, and smoking and it makes us happy. I will need a beer tonight once the second load of paving slabs has been unloaded.

In two days we will be heading home. There is no escape from that. It has to be done. I hope that I may be able to come back before too long but that depends on my treatment and how long I am signed off for, and all sorts of other unknowns, all of which contribute to a great deal of uncertainty. We cannot plan for the future because there are so many things that we do not know. That is a problem. It would be nice to be using this time to make plans. As it is, we can talk about maybes which is good too, but ultimately not completely satisfying. It adds a little to my uncertainty generally.

CHAPTER 16

LE CLOS DAVIAUD CHEZ MARTIN

I ought to explain a little about the house in France, given how big a role it is assuming.

In 2010 we had been on holiday in France, a little further north than the Charente – which is a region about two thirds of the way down France on the left. We had been staying in a villa with a pool. It was one of those holidays when the sun shines, the pool is there and all you really need to do from one day to the next is eat and swim and relax and sleep. We were happy.

One day we had arranged to meet someone in a local town and arrived slightly early. I wandered up to what turned out to be an estate agent and was soon transfixed by how much you could buy for how little money. I called Lucy over – 'Have you seen how cheap property is round here?'

I had not the slightest thought about actually buying somewhere. It was risky and spontaneous and I was a lawyer for goodness' sake – you don't make decisions on the spur of the moment.

Well, sometimes you do.

If you were to make a list of the qualities your dream French holiday house must have, they might include being near the coast and being within walking distance of a decent baker, bar, and restaurant. We have none of those. It is in the middle of nowhere.

It is built from a mix of clay and stones. It is finished with a pale cream render known locally as "*crepis*". The expansive roof is finished with Charente tiles of varying ages and hues – yellows, oranges and reds randomly spread around (the colours, that is, rather than the tiles themselves which are in vaguely symmetrical straight lines). And every window and door has the classic French wooden shutters painted in the traditional pale greeny-blue colour. The décor is fairly basic, with a woodburner in the kitchen and a huge fire place dominating the lounge. The flooring is a mix of wood and tiles.

What you really notice when you walk in the front door is the familiar smell that only exists there and a sense in which the house is reaching out its arms and hugging you in a welcoming embrace – 'You are meant to be here,' it seems to be saying, "*bienvenue*".

As important as the house, however, is the surrounding land and outbuildings. There are several fields left to grassland and four small animal enclosures, each with an animal hut in the middle. One day I hope to have them occupied again – the whiteboard in the kitchen has a shopping list that includes a pig, a donkey, hens, a goat, geese, and possibly a horse. Near the pond is a donkey shed nestling in some trees.

The house is on the top of a hill and, beyond our plot, the land continues to slope away into a valley and rises up again the other side, so we have a sense of space, a sense that exists whichever way one looks out. You have to make an effort to see another house. Sometimes a herd of friendly and inquisitive cows will graze the fields surrounding us – light brown in colour, paling to cream in the height of summer. They provide some company and interaction when human contact is sparse, or else feels too much.

At the front of the house is a swimming pool and terrace and we spend much of our time there. There is an old bread oven which I have partially restored, and which now serves as a pizza oven and is part of a large covered eating area I built.

Behind the house is a substantial barn. This houses a wood store, my workshop, a number of potting sheds, and some animal pens.

The sun rises across the valley and nothing interrupts our view of its passage across the sky until it sets on the far side, still with nothing but a few trees obscuring the view. At night it seems like you can see the universe. The light contamination is minimal (and mostly under our direct control) so it takes little effort to switch out all light and experience the blackness and the vast expanse – with shooting stars, satellites, space stations, and stars your only companion. When storms come – as they do regularly through the summer as the temperature and humidity build – one can see them building and approaching from miles away and watch as they hit or skirt the house and move on.

Mostly we stay on campus. The pool, football, cricket, table tennis, countless varieties of hide-and-seek, the trampoline and, more recently lounging around being teenagers, is enough for the kids, and for me there is a constant supply of maintenance and creation.

Aside from our dog, Roxy, and the local farm animals, there is much wildlife. There are nests all over the place. Songbirds of all shapes, sizes, and colours busy about from March to well into the autumn. Birds of prey soar and swoop. A barn owl roosted for a couple of years around the back of the house. Lizards sunbathe throughout the summer and keep warm behind shutters at night and in the winter, often sharing the space in winter with hibernating bats. Frogs keep a chorus going from dawn until well after human bedtime, save for the coldest months. There are, it being France, too many wasps and some giant ones that might be hornets and might not. We have bees nesting in the barn and once, when I arrived shortly after a snow fall, there were tracks around the house that could only have been from a wild boar, which are apparently plentiful in the surrounding countryside.

Inside the house there are mice – it is their house when we are not there, I think. And something lives in the extensive loft space. We have never seen it, only heard it, and can find no signs of it in the loft. We are, however, reliably and repeatedly assured by the locals that it is a pine martin – appropriate really.

Finally, tucked at the back of the house within the structure of the house, surrounded on three sides by wall, under the main roof, but open to the fields and countryside on one side, is quite possibly the best place to be in the entire world. It is peaceful there, surrounded with foliage and birdsong. It is cool in the heat of summer and everyone, dog or human, spends some part of their day in its tranquillity and peace.

It was there that Lucy and I would sit that first week in February in the evening, looking out across our new estate, drinking a glass of local Pineau, exhausted from whatever work we had been doing to kit the house out, and dreaming of possibilities.

In short, the house is a constant delight and source of fascination.

All of this contrasts so vividly with our lives in London. There it often feels like humans have sterilised the landscape, cleansed it of nature, and filled it with our detritus. In France, one has the strong sense of living with nature, of having taken a small space for ourselves (which we still share with many animal residents) while leaving most to whatever wants to be there. If we were to leave, nature would very soon reclaim it all. Humans dictate the speed and rhythm of London life, which seems to be ever faster. The pace of life in our corner of France has not changed for centuries, forever perhaps, dictated by the seasons and by the natural cycle of life. One can breathe, and that hug that the house gives when you first arrive gently slows your pace and brings you back to that cycle. The worries and stress of London life are dissolved. It feels right to be there.

Often when I am driving back up France to return to London, I can feel that stress re-entering me. Jobs, the to-do lists, the worries, start slowing coming back into my head as if I am re-entering another me, and rueing the one I am leaving behind.

CHAPTER 17

RETURN TO ENGLAND

Monday 5th September (Morning)

So here we are back in England. The last couple of days in France were anxious, but I filled them with packing and cleaning, and so distracted myself. There were times, however, when only a hug from someone would do. The journey home went smoothly and fairly quickly. We shared the driving and it was fine. There was the odd feeling of fear in me, getting on for panic at times, but nothing too severe or long-lasting.

We got back Friday night and, first thing Saturday, went off to my parents' 50th wedding anniversary. There was a mass, followed by a reception at their local pub. I had a reading to do at the mass, which went fine, and I felt okay with it. When we arrived at the pub, Lucy thought she had left her sunglasses at the church so I drove back, quite glad of the excuse to be able to put off a little longer the prospect of talking to family and old faces, long forgotten, about this and that. I got quite shaky doing that but had composed myself by the time I got back to the pub where things were already in full swing. I chatted happily to various people and felt alright. Indeed, various people apparently commented to Lucy that I seemed very well. I did feel that I was putting on a show. This was Mum and Dad's occasion and I did not want to distract from them.

There was certainly fear of going to the event. I did not know what people knew about what had been happening to me. I did not want to be the centre of attention or to distract from the main event. It is difficult to know what to say when people you have not seen for 20 years ask you how you are doing. Do you give them a potted history of the last 20 years or tell them just what the last few months have been like? What do they really want to hear? I found that by talking to a small number of groups of people one could gauge what was appropriate and found myself saying quite a lot about the last few months, as well as the last 20 years, and found a great deal of sympathy, as well as quite a number of similar stories.

When we got back, I was exhausted. I slept for two hours on the sofa and, even when I woke, I was good for nothing. All I was able to do was sit and watch TV.

Sunday was again difficult. I felt as if the haze from the dark days before the Priory was setting in again. I felt numb and as if there were a thick glass wall between me and the world. It was not quite as bad as those early days, however, because I was able to make a list of things to do and then do them. While Lucy took Gina and Jude off on an outing I sorted out the house and got the kids' things ready for going back to school. At various times I needed a hug of support and reassurance from Steph, which was gladly given and received.

Today so far has been hard. It is Gina's first day at senior school, so very exciting for that. Although still looking like a little girl in her too-big-for-her new uniform, surrounded at the gate by loads of much bigger girls, Gina was being very brave and grown-up and did not want us fussing round her. She had been here before for induction, knew what she was doing, and was quite happy to find her own way thank you very much. Good for her, although one of those rites of passage moments for us as we see our second child making that huge step up towards greater independence.

After dropping Gina off we walked into town to get a coffee. Road repairmen were sawing paving stones and the noise sent me *into shakes and severe anxiety. A siren from a passing ambulance did the same. It was scary just sitting and being.*

So why am I feeling like I am? We have done a lot – loads of cleaning at the house in France, the journey home, the stress of the reading and everything else at the 50th anniversary do. But I think it is more than that. Term is starting. People are going back to work. I watch it all happen and am not part of it. Our garden, decent sized by local standards, feels hemmed in. We live in a small box surrounded by other people, their builders, their noise and confusion. That great long period away that promised, and to a large extent delivered, so much is over. I am back now and need to face up to whatever is coming, and I do not feel able to do it and do not want to do it.

I was content and largely stable in France. I felt at ease, comfortable in my surroundings. Here I am ill at ease and scared. I jump at the slightest sound, even Lucy throwing shoes out from under the bed to find the right pair for Saturday's "do" made me shake with fear. And it takes time to get back in to what small routine I can manage. I could not find my medication until late on Saturday. So that was unnerving. I wanted to meditate this morning but had to find the iPod and it was not charged. All these little things just accentuate the change between France and here. They will get sorted and I will re-establish some control and routine, but right now it is hard.

On the way back from getting a haircut I stopped and sat on a park bench and felt like one of the characters from Larkin's 'Toads Revisited', for whom it did not suit "being one of the men you meet of an afternoon, palsied old step takers, hair eyed clerks with the jitters, wax fleshed outpatients still vague from accidents or characters in long coats deep in the litter baskets, all dodging the Toad work by being stupid or weak." I feel like one of that band but am not sure which character's shoes fit me best.

Thursday 8th September

Just back from seeing the psychiatrist, my first contact with the medical profession for five weeks or so. This was preceded by a trip to casualty with Lucy, who has hurt her foot, and taking two of the kids to the orthodontist yesterday, which was significant on various levels. First, I was able to do it, to be the responsible adult, reassure them, make decisions about their treatment, and liaise with the dentist and all that. Secondly, it showed how Lucy, the kids and I trusted me to do it.

I wasn't too bad for most of the journey to London. I deliberately had a book to read to distract myself, but getting to the ticket turnstile at Bank was more intense. I found myself heading up the travellator shaking and hugging myself close and kind of bowing over, cowering. Since then I have found my arms shaking at various times.

I gave the doctor an overview of the last few weeks. I mentioned the suicidal thoughts while away, the episodes of seizure-type things, general improvement, still being very tired, a lack of libido, problems with disturbed sleep, managing to cope with things like the dentist and the 50th anniversary. I emphasised how happy and calm I was generally while away.

His view, not surprisingly, is that I am making good progress. I am clearly better than I was, and he reckons I am slightly ahead of the norm, although he probably says that to everyone. I asked him how he would describe me to a fellow psychiatrist and he said a case of anxiety and depression with a number of interesting complications who is making good solid progress. He said that people do not progress in a straight, or even standard curve or line, but rather with a series of ups and downs and it is mapping the overall direction of travel that counts. I asked about timescales which I know he cannot be definite about. He said not to think about work for a couple of months more but that he would expect me to be ready to go back within 12 months or so.

He wants me to start psychotherapy ASAP, to stay off work as aid and to double my meds to 40mg of citalopram a day. And he wants to see me again in two weeks' time.

Monday 12th September (Afternoon)

Another Monday. The kids all go off to school, the grown-ups in other houses go off to work, and I stay here.

I have a plan for today, finishing off some garden clearance followed by a trip to the tip, but after today I will have nothing to do. I will have to find another way to fill my time, another way to get me out of bed, another way to give me some feeling of contribution, achievement, purpose. I almost want to drag out the end of today's work, maybe do the tip tomorrow, but no.

I do take Lucy for a coffee to get her up and out of the house as she has not been out for a couple of days and is threatening to spend the day in bed by the look of things, but in reality, I need to get it done. The feeling of failing to complete my task is for the moment worse than the fear of what tomorrow does not hold, and the day after that, and the day after that.

I had a sense of purpose when I came back from the psychiatrist – appointments to make, people to update and all that, but it did not last long. The appointments are all in the diary and I must wait for them to come along. I am desperate for the therapy to start to inject some momentum to my treatment.

Friday was tired and so is today. I think it is a combination of activity, physical work in the garden, as well as being busy for most of the time, a late night on Saturday, and the responsibility for not being looked after so much. I am quite anxious and quite depressed. I feel flat, numb. The leaves are coming off the trees and soon the branches will be bare and ready for winter. I feel that too, although of course clearing up the leaves will give me something to do in the garden.

That feeling of the world going back to school and work in September without me was really strong. Until then I could convince myself that I had had a couple of months off work followed by a long holiday in the summer. As everyone else went back to their real lives, however, at the start of a new school year, I felt my absence from that acutely – that I was not ready to join them. I knew I wasn't, but the seriousness of my continuing illness was reinforced. The strangeness was intensified by Lucy not working at the time either so that the kids all left the house to go about their business and engage with the world outside while the grown-ups stayed home – an odd role reversal.

I needed things to occupy me and give me a sense of purpose. I had proved in France that manual labour was good on many counts – not taxing mentally, mindful in the sense that you could keep your attention focused on the task in hand, exercise, and a sense of achievement. The garden project was a good place to start.

I had always enjoyed gardening. It was a decent-size plot for South-West London, most of which I had replanted over the years. There were a number of bushes that were now mature and which should have been getting some serious pruning attention through the spring and summer but which had been neglected in my illness and were now overgrown, cutting out light, smothering each other, and killing an old tree.

I decided that I would cut all the big bushes right back to their base. I was confident that they were healthy and would grow back in due course, but that by allowing light to penetrate down to the soil again we might allow all sorts of other things to spring up which had previously not had a chance. Equally, as the mature bushes regrew I would take time to make sure they gave each other space, were kept to a manageable size and did not become too dominant or stifling. I started at the end nearest the house, creating huge piles of garden debris as I went.

Half way down on the left was a Pyracantha. Now these are impressive ladies – they must be feminine with that ending right? They grow tall and strong, with thick branches and glossy green leaves. Their upper branches will spread for several feet, well over our garden in one direction and over the neighbour's in the other. Their branches are festooned with two-inch long thorns which will rip through clothing without much effort, and through skin without any at all. They are not to be messed with.

For most of the year they sit there proud and tall, watching while all the other plants do their flowering thing, competing with each other for attention. Then, when everyone else is tiring and fading, starting the gradual decline to winter, but holding out as long as possible to gather as much of the sun's precious energy as they can to replenish their roots, the Pyracantha does her thing and clothes herself from head to toe in gaudy but irresistibly attractive orange or red berries. They hang in vast bunches beckoning every bird in the district to come and feast. It is the garden's last glorious hurrah.

It was autumn now and there was no way that I was going to deprive the Pyracantha of her few weeks of glory and so I passed on by, determining to return once the remaining berries had turned to brown.

Later that evening I sat on a bench with a hard-earned beer, admiring my labour. I reflected on how my efforts seemed a telling metaphor for what had happened to nearly every aspect of my life over the last several months. I had stopped work, stopped being a school governor, stopped going to church and all the duties I had acquired connected to it, and much else besides. I hoped that I would return to levels of greater activity and engagement with the world in due course, but for now they were cut right back.

When they returned I would endeavour to control them better, prevent them from overpowering everything else, and in the meantime I would have a chance to see what else might flourish, now that their domineering shade had been removed. Inevitably that led me to reflect on the Pyracantha and what it represented, if all the other parts of my life had been cut back. It was some months before I returned my attention to it, by which time Lucy and I had agreed to spend some time apart. I cut it back to its base.

CHAPTER 18

FINDING SOMETHING TO DO

Monday 12th September (Continued)

I am going to try to find a course – carpentry or something else practical. It will not tax my brain but will give me something to do, use the time constructively, and perhaps give me some skills to use at a later date in France or somewhere else. It will also give me a routine, a purpose. Being signed off for a further two months has had a big effect on me. It will take me almost to the end of my six months' sick pay. It underlines how ill I have been and does not leave me long after that to decide what then happens – what do I do, where we live and all that.

We had always had a substantial mortgage on the house. Believing my lawyer's income would continue, we had financed the purchase of the house in France by increasing that mortgage. With sick pay running out, no clarity of when, or if, I would be able to return to work, and in what capacity, and Lucy keen to make changes, to do something, we had begun to think about selling the house and finding something smaller so as to reduce the financial pressure.

Monday 19th September (Morning)

Monday again. The kids have all gone to school. There is, as in any house, a routine to this now. Steph gets herself up before seven. My alarm goes off at seven. I listen to the radio for a few minutes (on the mornings when Lucy does not shout at me to turn it off the moment she hears those nice voices from the Today programme). At around 7.12am I heave myself out of bed, see Steph cleaning her teeth and wander upstairs to wake up Gina, who is always cross about being woken up. I then go down to make tea for me and Lucy, take her cup to her in bed and then go in and wake Jude.

By now Steph has left the house to a chorus of goodbyes. Jude is always awake when I go in, or dozing at least, and we normally play some silly game by way of a wake-up ritual. Then it's breakfast for Gina, Jude, and me, bundle Gina out the door, and at some stage Lucy will stagger downstairs, limping with her bad leg.

Yesterday we took the kids into Central London as part of the Open House weekend. We went round Parliament which was good, then wandered up Whitehall, had some lunch and then tried to get into the Supreme Court and the Abbey, but both were closed by then. We did see troops filing out of the Abbey after the Battle of Britain memorial service, and a fly past by a single Spitfire or Hurricane. There was also the London stage of the Tour of Britain bike ride, so various streets were cordoned off for the event.

It was my idea to do it and I was pleased we did. I did not mention it to anyone the day before in case I did not feel up to it on the day; but I did, and everyone wanted to go, and we did it and it was good. I was a bit tired and anxious by the end – ordering lunch in Pret a Manger was a bit touch-and-go at one point – and I shouted at Gina and Jude who insisted on fighting in the car on the way home. I threatened to get out and wait until they were quiet.

Saturday was busy – watching Jude play football first thing, then something I can't remember, then looking at a house, then people looking at this one, then my senior partner round here and then supper and drinks with the neighbours. I really did not want to go. I was knackered. But Lucy persuaded me and I stayed for a couple of hours and coped, and put on a good show, I think, before running out of steam and coming home. I was in bed by 10.00, a good half-hour before Lucy came home with the kids. I am now worried that I cannot remember the names of any of the people there, which will be slightly embarrassing when I meet them in the street.

My senior partner was very kind, gentle, and encouraging. We talked a bit about work, the comings and goings etc., which was okay. A couple of the cases I had been working on before I left have been reported in the press, which he mentioned. He reassured me that he had always thought it would take six months for me to recover, that I should not give up hope of getting well enough to return, into whatever role, that I was missed etc. He does make it all seem possible, and much less frightening. Also, as we carry on looking at houses and do not find anything, we realise how much we like this one and that requires me to be earning the current type of salary which probably does mean staying where I am. Who knows?

I have been trying to do something every day, seeing friends, exercise. The higher dose of the pills, however, is having a big effect on me. I think I am a little less anxious although it is not gone entirely by any means. But I am exhausted. Every day I am sleeping for a couple of hours during the day. And I can feel myself grinding to a halt some days, and Lucy can see it in my face and she sends me off to bed.

Today I am feeling brave. I am going to take the dog on the train to Kingston with my bike and then we are going to cycle down to Windsor – 20 odd miles or so – then get the train back. I am waiting for the trains to go off-peak so I can take my bike. I have packed lunches for me and the dog, something for me to read while she has a rest somewhere along the route, water for us both, and bowls for her. It feels like an adventure and I hope I am not over-committing myself.

Tuesday 20th September (Morning)
There was a degree of slight nervousness about the whole bike ride expedition – is this too much, I am responsible for me and for the dog, will it be too long for the dog etc? My plan is to ride as far as seems sensible, but no further than Windsor. I know there is a train back, but I have not checked how often it runs, or where it comes back to, so there are various unknowns which create their

own anxiety and uncertainty. I also struggle to hold many things in my head at any one time, which perhaps explains the slight lack of planning.

Anyway, we take a train to Kingston where we disembark. I am on the wrong side of the river for the path but, once I have crossed the bridge, I can set off. Three miles to Hampton Court, 24 miles to Windsor.

Roxy is fresh and running well. I cycle with her off the lead and she runs at my side generally, but will often detour to explore a smell or drink from a puddle.

We bound along at a steady 10 or 11 miles per hour following the great bend right in the river, and soon see the chimneys of Hampton Court Palace. You arrive on the Richmond side of the river and then the path switches to the other side of the river so we cross the bridge and carry on.

We pass where my cousins and then my granny used to live in East Molesey, just off the river. Walton is where my mum worked for many years and beyond that is Weybridge where I used to go to school. The route is fairly empty. There are some runners, walkers, and cyclists, but the path is wide and it is easy to pass them or be passed.

And then we get to the ferry across the Thames at Weybridge.

It is a wonderful set-up. There is a sign explaining that you must summon the ferry with the bell, but only on the quarter hours, and a list of fares. I assume that the ferryman will want to fill his boat and there is only me here, so I guess I will have to wait. I look at my watch – 25 past. Should I wait for half past? I decide to risk it and break the rules. I give the bell a good ring and see a man on the other side stop his repair work on a boat and wander over to a small, open-topped boat and make the short crossing over to me. I persuade the dog in, heave the bike in too and pay the man the £3 he requests – I am sure the sign said £4.50 but I am not going to quibble.

The crossing takes less than a minute. He explains where to go on the other side and off we go.

Aside from the two bar-girls in the pubs I stop at later for coffees, and the hellos to people I pass, this is the only human contact I have all day and it is very pleasant. He is warm and seems very happy, and certainly very keen to help me.

We make our way along paths that are sometimes grassy, sometimes gravel or even tarmac. There are locks every now and then where the signs say I have to dismount and the dog has to be on a lead. There are always pleasure boats waiting to go through, or in the process of going through, and a lock keeper's cottage with fine displays of flowers. I am reminded of hours spent as a child at a lock near us watching, and sometimes helping, the boats through. It was my place to escape to, my little idyll of peace and calm.

We pass numerous birds – ducks, geese, and swans, this year's cygnets still a little brown but well on the way to their splendid Dulux white. Three herons fly off in front of us at different moments during the day and at various points there are lines of 50 or more ducks and geese standing on the bank who all jump into the water in turn at our approach, like collapsing dominos. At one point where I get the route wrong and we have to retrace our steps, we manage to dislodge a good 80 or so birds, first from one direction and then, once they have had time to regain their perch and pecking order, and I have had time to realise we are on the wrong route, from the other.

One would think the route would be fairly easy – stick next to the big wet thing and you should be okay. But at various points, private fields, playgrounds, houses, and waterworks mean the path turns inland. At Chertsey Bridge something makes me think that the path must be crossing to the other bank, so I take the lives of the three of us – me, the dog, and the bike – in my hands as we navigate the very narrow pavement over the bridge as traffic roars past oblivious.

But there is no path over the other side, only a pub with a couple of early drinkers in the garden. A lady tells me it is the other side, the side I was on, and so I repeat the dance with death crossing back over the bridge and recall the two facts I was meant to remember from my limited research on the internet – use the ferry at Weybridge and do not cross Chertsey Bridge – well I have now crossed it twice.

And so we go on, past Shepperton lock, through a meadow which comes right down to the river and is populated by enormous brown cows and their, by now, large calves. Somewhere we go under the M25 and are officially in the rest of England.

We lunch by a lovely stretch of river marred only by a road not far enough away from the bank. We stop there because it is time to rest, and also because I need a pee. We have our lunch, Roxy her biscuits and water, and me my sandwich. Roxy has been tiring a little. We have done 18 miles or so and her normal walk is about 7 so this is a long one. She has been running behind me for a few miles and I have slowed to allow her to keep up. She gratefully scoffs all her lunch and has a lie down. After 20 minutes or so she is completely revived – I ask her whether she wants a walk and she is barking and jumping madly at me, so I reckon she is okay to continue.

We travel on – a big detour round Datchet or Old Windsor and before I know it, or expect it, I see the spires of the Eton college chapel and then Windsor Castle itself. It is almost an anti-climax. We are done, we have arrived and it is over.

I stop at a pub and have a coffee and read my book for a bit, and then walk to the train station. I am relieved to see that the train back stops at Putney, where, after heaving the bike and dog up the stairs, we walk up Putney hill and then cycle home across the common. Roxy has enough energy left to chase the trains as we take the footbridge over the tracks at the end of our road, and we are home.

It feels like a great achievement. A day out, on my own, slightly risky in the sense of being on my own and having to make decisions and dealing with the unknown. There was anxiety for sure at the start, but generally I coped well. It felt deeply mindful, focused only on the route and the nature we travelled through. I left behind all worries about how I was, about the family, jobs to do, the future. And I felt happy, at peace, in a way I had not felt, in London at least, for a long, long time.

I am tired when I get back, but also energised and empowered by the achievement in a strange way. By way of example, the phone rings. Lucy says it is a call she is expecting and answers it, but it is someone asking for me. Guessing that it is someone trying to sell something she is only too pleased to put me on and it is British Gas wanting our custom back from Southern Electric. Rather than do my normal, which is to panic a lot and then say we are happy with our current supplier, I engage in 30 minutes of discussion with the nice chap before we both conclude that we are probably better off with Southern or that the savings, if any, to be gained from switching are so small as not to be worth it. But I do also decide to call Southern to check on our current deal and have 45 minutes of chat with them, give them updated readings from the meters, discuss prices and packages and negotiate a refund of £700 of credit we have built up, reduced monthly payments, and a new deal.

All of which is stuff that I can scarcely cope with when well but for some reason have the patience and energy and peace of mind to deal with now. So, there is a great example perhaps of one achievement giving me the courage and confidence to deal with others.

In addition, in the midst of my negotiations for power supply, Lucy gets an email from an agent who wants to take her on with her new book, which is great news and I have the presence of mind to put some Prosecco on ice to celebrate with her. That may not sound that much, but feeling the excitement for her, being able to show it and responding to it appropriately, are things that were not possible for me a few weeks ago.

This morning, I should say, I am yawning a lot and my legs are tired. The neighbour kindly offers to walk the dog and I settle down to write this entry, and prepare for my first one-to-one CBT session since going into the Priory.

Re-engaging with therapy was important and I was eager to build on what I had learnt and understood in group sessions in the Priory. The time in France, although beneficial in many ways, felt like a holiday from the work of trying to sort my head out and get me back to a point where I could start to re-engage with the outside world. My psychiatrist had recommended CBT, with the same person I had seen briefly before I went into the Priory. I was happy to go along *with whatever he suggested. I saw her in the same Harley Street clinic in which I sometimes saw him – he practices out of various places so where I saw him would depend on the day of the week. Sometimes, therefore, I would bump into him when I was seeing her and vice versa. It lent a medical tone to the therapy sessions.*

CBT is primarily focused on the here-and-now, how you experience circumstances and events now, why and, where appropriate, challenging the basis of unhelpful reactions and thought patterns. The traditionally short-term nature of CBT means that a lot of the work has to be undertaken by the patient or client outside the sessions. In addition, because the focus is on changing long-held patterns of thought / feeling / action, you need to do a lot of practice – it is not going to get fixed by an hour once a week in some secluded therapy room, but has to be repeated over and over in the real world.

Some of this homework can be recording events and your feelings, thoughts and reactions. Sometimes you may be asked to identify particular episodes and analyse them in greater detail, breaking them down in the same way one might do in a session with the therapist. There may also be exercises around doing things or going to places that you have been avoiding or are scared of, trying to break down in a gradual and controlled way some of the demons that surround them.

For a week, I was tasked with keeping a detailed diary of how I spent my time every day, breaking the day down into two-hour slots, from early morning until last thing at night, recording what I was doing but also including the anticipated feelings I associated with the activity and then the actual feelings. The primary focus of the work was my anxiety. Anxiety, by its very nature, is largely anticipatory in nature. This record therefore would allow me to reflect on and challenge the basis of anticipated feelings and also compare them with how things actually turned out.

One particular incident from that week is still raw in my mind. Tuesday was the day the bin men came, first thing in the morning, albeit waiting politely until the local fox population had been through the bags to check for anything tasty. That meant the bins had to be put out on Monday night.

In those days, we had to sort the recycling into different categories – cardboard, glass, plastic and tins. Then there was the food waste and general rubbish. It does not sound that complicated right? Because it wasn't. But halfway through, the anxiety that had been building up around it from no obvious source got the better of me and I collapsed on the ground in tears, unable to cope with the situation and unable to cope with my inability to cope, if that makes sense. I was shaking convulsively, tears pouring down my cheeks, utterly helpless and distraught – over the recycling for goodness' sake. I was helped to bed by one of the kids while the others finished the job.

CHAPTER 19

GETTING OUT AND ABOUT

Wednesday 28th September

I am on the train to Manchester as I write, to stay with my brother, Andy, and his partner. The trip has come about because Lucy has said she feels trapped and stifled with me around and needs a break and wants me out of the house. Andy has often said I am welcome there. I think the two of them must have spoken as well because he renewed his offer just as she was saying why don't I go and stay with him. I don't really mind whether they did or didn't ... except it does make me a bit cross. I am trying hard; generally looking after myself, keeping myself busy or out of the way, doing lots with the kids, and my fair share of housework. I am sure that it is not easy living with someone who is at the same time both very anxious, while also, more generally, emotionally flat. The drugs, while taking the edge off the anxiety are, at the same time, numbing my emotions. It is also strange for us to be spending so much time together in each other's pockets, neither of us having jobs to go to outside the house. The strain is showing.

There is a princess falling asleep on the seat across the aisle from me, her face turned to me, so that, unfortunately for her, I will be the first thing she sees when she opens her eyes.

I saw both my therapist and psychiatrist yesterday. He is worried that I am still getting anxiety problems despite my medication and the passage of time. He could dose me up further, but he would end up tranquilising me and does not want to. He is thinking about whether he could give me something else to take as and when I need it, which might help but sounds a bit dangerous. I thought about taking an overdose last night, and about jumping under the train today. Not serious planning but the thoughts crossing my mind about the options. Would having more drugs to hand make that worse?

My therapist wants to do some trauma-like therapy involving eye movement to address my issues around beatings at home. Some, at least, of my anxiety moments are around worrying about getting things right, finding the right cleaning product in the supermarket as requested by Lucy, sorting out the rubbish. It may be that underlying it is a fear that if I do not get it right then I will be beaten. I do feel constantly liable to account for myself. As my therapist put it, that may have been originally down to others, but now I have taken over the duty of scaring myself shitless. The beatings now are not physical and are not administered by a third party, but are equally effective in keeping me on my toes and in a state of constant threat.

The Pendolino train is doing its magic trick with rivers and lakes on the track side tilted up at angles without the water all falling out. Quite amazing. Engineers would tell me that it is an optical illusion caused by the train tilting and my brain not being used to that and so assuming the train is flat and the ground tilted. But that is not nearly as much fun, and does not explain how my brain can be content with the conclusion, based on its observations, that rivers and lakes are indeed defying the basic principles of gravity.

Battery is running low on the laptop so will stop there and read my book and wait for the sleeping beauty to open her eyes and kiss me ...

Saturday 1st October
She didn't ...

Have had a very nice few days with Andy and his partner. I felt very little anxiety while there, no shaking, no fears. I jumped at the odd dog barking and at a car crash in a film I watched at the cinema, *but otherwise nothing really. I was a little more on edge with her than with him because I don't know her as well, and comfortable silences are more difficult with people you don't know well, so you end up thinking you have to fill them, or worrying about what the other person is thinking about the fact that you are not saying anything. Or at least I do anyway. But she is very gentle and kind. We walked together on Friday and also spent a couple of hours gardening.*

He is quite particular about food. What to eat, when. It has to be just right, right for the weather, for the time of day, made from just the right ingredients with the best possible utensils and with all possible care. It means that they eat really well. Often that indecision, worrying, questioning, would affect me. It kind of washed over me this time. I found it very easy not to make any decisions, or at least not many, and those I did have to make involved no great effort or stress.

We were pretty active. I took myself to the cinema when I arrived to fill the time before Andy finished work. We did a couple of decent bike rides. Friday was walking and gardening and then gathering wood for a school project Andy is running on Monday. I marvel at their ability to vary plans to suit how they are feeling. On one of the days we skipped the planned gardening because she was hungover and reckoned the bending down would do bad things to her head, and on another we stop some wood collecting before we are properly finished because it is too hot. If it were down to me I would feel obliged to soldier on, get it done. They are kind to themselves, and also calm and content.

Packing for home made me a little anxious, which was the only time. I don't know whether it was the worry of getting everything in the bag, the anticipation of stress on the journey, or of going home. I think I want to go home but it is hard to feel strongly about things. I don't want to feel that I have to stay away from home, to exclude myself or to be excluded. I also miss the kids and Lucy.

Sunday 9th October 2011

It is Sunday evening and X Factor was meant to be on, so I was going to catch up with you, Diary, but Jude could not find his school bag, Gina said she saw it at school and did not think to tell anyone and then she could not find jeans and everyone started shouting so there is no X Factor and they have all been sent to bed. I tried to avoid the stress of the fracas by washing up, but in the end thought it was unfair to Lucy, and perhaps the kids, to leave them at it, working themselves into ever more of a frenzy so, with a deep breath, I ventured forth. So now the kids are going to bed, Lucy is doing Spanish homework and I have snatched a few minutes.

A lot has happened in a week. I think the trip to Manchester, although tiring because of being active both physically and alcoholically, did me the world of good. I came home feeling calmer and more confident. It also did Lucy a load of good too so that she was pleased to have me back.

Lucy is challenging me to do things and to stop relying on her so much. Last Sunday we were invited to some friends for a barbecue. I was reluctant when the call came to invite us, but I think Lucy agreed without telling me. I forgot about it for most of the day but then felt very agitated on the way round there. Lucy talked to me firmly, said I should go in, that she was not going to go in alone, she wanted to be doing things with me. So, I went in and she kept an eye out for me and I survived. And that helped Lucy feel better about me – that I was making an effort for her I guess and, indeed, for myself.

Similarly, last night we were invited to one of her friend's 45th birthday with a load of people she knows quite well, and I, only a little. I felt tired and shaky. I had gone for a sleep at half past seven and woke at half past eight to go to the party and you do always feel crap when waking from a daytime sleep, so she tells me. So, I did not want to go, but I agreed, and had a fantastic time. I chatted to various people, often without Lucy; we even danced together for the first time in ages. We ended up being the last to leave at half past two. It left me tired today but was a great sign of what you can do if you try, and you face down your anxiety.

There is a contrast between listening to your body and doing what it tells you – for example, when you are tired, don't go out – and the contrary exhortation to break cycles of negative, depressive behaviour. A CBT approach to my reluctance to be sociable might have been to say that you think you are not sociable, and that you will not be able to manage. As a result, you feel unsociable and anxious about the party and so you do not go. This then reinforces the initial thoughts and feelings, creating a negative cycle which will repeat itself over and over if left unchecked. A CBT approach would say, you may not feel like going to the party, but, as your homework, just go. By breaking the cycle, you encourage more positive thoughts and feelings. Lucy just likes parties so that was her argument. In any event, I went, had a lovely time, realised people did like me, and that I could engage with them in some degree of confidence.

In therapy, I have started EMDR[1] which seemed to have some effect. My therapist had me get into the memories and feelings of being beaten as a kid, as graphically as I could, and I felt the anger and fear inside me. Then as I closed my eyes she gently tapped her fingers on my hands and I felt myself calm down. It is the first of several sessions, but it seemed to have a positive effect, even if I have no idea how.

[1] EMDR stands for Eye Movement Desensitisation and Reprocessing therapy. On its website, the EMDR Association of the UK and Ireland describes the therapy as follows, better than any description I could attempt:

When a person is involved in a distressing event, they may feel overwhelmed and their brain may be unable to process the information like a normal memory. The distressing memory seems to become frozen on a neurological level. When a person recalls the distressing memory, the person can re-experience what they saw, heard, smelt, tasted or felt, and this can be quite intense. Sometimes the memories are so distressing, the person tries to avoid thinking about the distressing event to avoid experiencing the distressing feelings.

Some find that the distressing memories come to mind when something reminds them of the distressing event, or sometimes the memories just seem to just pop into mind. The alternating left-right stimulation of the brain with eye movements, sounds or taps during EMDR, seems to stimulate the frozen or blocked information processing system.

In the process the distressing memories seem to lose their intensity, so that the memories are less distressing and seem more like "ordinary" memories. The effect is believed to be similar to that which occurs naturally during REM sleep (Rapid Eye Movement) when your eyes rapidly move from side to side. EMDR helps reduce the distress of all the different kinds of memories, whether it was what you saw, heard, smelt, tasted, felt or thought.

I struggled through Gina's school concert – it was a house competition so there were mostly kids in the audience who were allowed to make as much noise as they wanted between performances which was really distressing. Then we had to face a very crowded bar area at the interval where you are nose-to-nose with a bunch of people you don't know, and everyone is moving in totally different directions holding three glasses of wine each. I was saved by Jude who was not feeling too good and so I could take him home.

I am walking or running with dogs every day which means I have a routine and gives me time on my own as well as exercise. I often stop for a coffee at a café and, although the caffeine is welcome, I tend to end up feeling very down and flat sitting there. I do not know if it is all the other people there talking to each other, or the realisation that I am there because I cannot do my job, or what, but it always brings me down a bit. I tend to recover when I head off again and feel better for the caffeine fix.

We spent Saturday afternoon over at the school across the road on a community action day which was fun, painting the front door, gardening, painting the school gate, that sort of thing. There were a group of 25 or so and it felt good to be part of the team, part of the community, doing something good for the world.

When I realised I was painting the front door, and that every visitor or child, parent or staff that came into the building for the next several years would be confronted with my handiwork, it did make me take a little more care than I might otherwise have done. I used to be a governor there, having stopped at the start of the year when, in hindsight, things were getting on top of me and Lucy was concerned about the lack of time I spent with the family – when I did come home at a sensible time it was in order to go a governors' meeting. She was right and looking back it was just one of a number of things that were not in proportion and were making me over-worked, over-stretched and under-nurtured. I do not miss it for a minute although I know I did make a contribution when I was there. I am happy now to make my contribution with a paint brush.

Wednesday 11ᵗʰ October

Forgot my brother Pete's birthday, or at least I remembered a few days in advance and made a mental note to buy a card and send it off but my problem is that there is no reliable place to store mental notes so it went disregarded until the day itself. I could not face a nasty garage card and concluded that at 5.30pm it was not so important that I had to rush to WH Smiths immediately etc. – a sense of proportion? Surely not. Anyway, I called him instead and had a nice chat. I had not spoken to him for a good while – several weeks if not more. I guess I had been avoiding it from a misplaced sense of fear, but it was nice to catch up.

Make yourself do the things you are putting off. Schedule them and then make sure you do them because they are not as bad as they seem, and even being able to tick them off and have that satisfaction is a reward in itself and one less thing to worry about, one less thing nagging at the back of your head.

I did the same with a call to my mum. That was nice for all the same reasons but then I talked about my EMDR therapy. I hesitated because of course the question would arise, if she thought about it, what were the traumatic events I was talking about? So, she did think about it and she asked whether I think a lot about my car crash. She thinks that might have been the start of all my problems.

Now, I did have a car crash, 'tis true. And it was a bit hairy. We wrote off a BMW estate. But it was only a five car shunt on the motorway (albeit the fast lane at night) and no one was hurt. I very rarely think about it at all save to bemoan the fact that I used to drive a 5 Series BMW which was exciting and now I drive a Ford Galaxy which just isn't, however much the black-out windows we inherited from the previous owner, make us look like drug dealers or pimps. I could not bring myself to tell her the reality of the trauma I am being required to revisit.

I had a further EMDR session on Tuesday. Back to the same image. Me, aged eight or something, sent upstairs to my bedroom by my mum to wait for my dad to arrive with his leather-soled slipper. I was to wait kneeling over the bed, trousers and pants down so he could arrive and administer the punishment. There would be no words spoken other than my shrieks of pain. He would hit me a number of times and then leave me to my tears. There was no attempt to contextualise it with my crime, whatever minor offence that may have been, no comfort afterwards, and no reconciliation or attempt to move forward. I would be expected to go downstairs at some time later with my face free of tears. There would be no discussion of what had happened.

So, there I am in therapy thinking about this scene and I see my dad with pointed ears and evil eyebrows – he does have quite wild ones anyway, but these were really wild. I was scared, angry, and ashamed all at the same time and was shaking in the therapy room. At times, I had images of wanting to hit him. And then there is a boy lying in bed afterwards, snivelling, scared, crying, alone, wanting to know he is loved but feeling very much like he isn't because one parent has done this to him and the other sentenced him to it in the full knowledge of what was to happen. And no one came to see him or comfort him.

And I see my adult self get into bed next to him and cuddle him to myself and then I do something I have not been able to do forever – a tear trickles down my face. I am crying for myself. I am comforting and reassuring and loving the little boy I was, and I can cry for him. And I can fight for him and beat the tormentor. And the funny thing is that in all of these images I am confused by images of me and Jude and the hugs and the reassurance and the love we give each other and express to each other which is a massive part of the relationship we have. At times, I do not know if I am really hugging myself or hugging him. As my therapist says at the end of the session – 'Good work today.'

Later that day, Jude came home ill from school. We gave him medicine to ease his pain and bring down the temperature. I put him to bed and wondered what to do next, except I knew just what to do as he is lying there crying, so I kicked off my shoes and climbed in next to him and for 20 minutes we lay there with his back to me while I held him tight and told him it was all going to be okay. And in time, it was.

I have never talked to my dad about him beating me. I have thought many times about doing so, but ours is not a relationship where that is an easy thing to contemplate, much less do. Through EMDR and other therapy I was able to understand the way in which my unconscious thinking patterns had been influenced by those experiences and how I had projected the fear they instilled onto other relationships, other people, other situations. And in that processing, I was able to forgive. I once read a definition that forgiveness means to stop wishing for a different past. I think that is true and I have come to accept that this is just what happened and it has, along with countless other experiences, good and bad, shaped me, and I can accept, and even like, who I am as a result. And, of course, the EMDR helped me understand that I no longer needed to fear him, or those other people onto whom I had projected those feelings of fear.

Although I have no understanding of the science behind it, the therapy seemed to enable me to revisit memories and re-evaluate them. They had been locked in my memory with particular meanings attached to them and it was as if I was able to step back into the actual memories and reassess the meanings and rules that had been attached to them and create new ones. Our unconscious brain works on rules, habits, that we build up over the years. Just as it takes time to create them, so it takes time to change them. Fear of authority figures, and the resulting desire to appease them, was a well-established rule my unconscious was quick to deploy. That does not change easily but I can recognise, if I am attentive, when I am replaying that rule and challenge it, by reference to my experiences in EMDR. I do not need to be physically afraid, or indeed afraid in any other way. My view, my needs, are as valid and as important as theirs and I do not need simply to bend to their will for my own safety.

My kids have also helped me understand a little of the anger I often feared in my dad. They tell me that the things that used to lead to me being angry now result in me being scared.

I think that a lot of anger is simply an expression of not feeling safe in a situation, and the fear that results creates a fight instinct which manifests itself as anger. When someone gets angry with us, there is often a tendency to respond in kind, whereas often a better response, if one can calm (or perhaps more accurately own) one's own feelings, is to respond with kindness towards this expression of huge discomfort, anxiety and fear, seek to understand it and to reassure the individual.

There are things you can do when not at work that you could never do otherwise. On Monday, I cycled with Steph to school and then went to pick her up on the bike too, so she could get used to the route and reassure herself about doing it – it was her idea to do it and it was so nice. One of those rites of passage moments in a way, because for me, the biggest thing about cycling to school, rather than being driven or taking the train or bus, and apart from the obvious dangers as well as the cold and the exercise, was the freedom, the independence it gives you. And to help her to take that independence was special.

The woodwork is coming on. One bedside table is done and another on the way. The second will be better, partly because I am more skilled with the tools and can copy the design. I have had lots of accolades for the first one, partly because they do not realise that lots of the funny marks are not just lovely, natural timber, but errors of different kinds.

There is something fantastically therapeutic about woodwork. It was something I started tinkering with in my mid-twenties. I attended an evening course and made the coffee table that the kids have grown up with and is still in Lucy's lounge. I made various shelves and a funky Teletubbies-style wardrobe for the kids when they were little. When we moved to our posh grown-up house we had a posh grown-up kitchen installed. After a year or two we were complaining about lack of storage space and there was a corner behind the door which would have been an ideal place for a tall unit to house mops and the vacuum cleaner and such like. And so I made one.

Carpentry cannot be rushed. It requires focus and care, is very much a mindful activity, and allows for creativity and expression. There is also something very soothing about working with the grain of the wood, planing, sanding, polishing, feeling its natural texture and strength.

CHAPTER 20

JUST BECAUSE I DO STUFF, DOESN'T MEAN I'M NOT ILL

I had, through work, a permanent health insurance policy which was designed to provide replacement income after my work sick pay ran out. It was now five months or so since I broke down. The sick pay would last another month, after which we would need to rely on the insurance. With the help of Lucy and the HR team at work I set about completing the lengthy claim form. With a physical injury or illness, I suspect that the process is relatively straightforward, based on medical evidence and opinion. You can see the injury or illness. It's less easy with mental illness. The only person who really knew what I was suffering was me. How do you persuade a stranger who you never meet that you are too ill to work? And there is always the nagging doubt in your own judgement too.

I had certainly improved from my lowest points and was trying to be active because that is what my psychiatrist was recommending, but he and I both knew that I was a long way away from being well enough to return to work. And everything about the prospect of returning to my work terrified me. The insurers, at various times, sought to argue that in fact I had *decided* not to return to my old work, that this was a lifestyle choice on my part, not anything to do with my illness.

For my part, over the coming months and years, I did come to the conclusion that I did not want to try to return to my old job, but that was because I did not feel that I could, that it would evoke just too much anxiety. On a very few occasions I did have to go to the office to meet with HR and every time I was paralysed with fear and in floods of tears before, during, and after the visit.

There was also this confusing contrast between wanting desperately to get better, doing as much as possible to progress that, while every now and then, when the insurer wanted to review my cover, having to argue how ill I still was, and how incapable I was of returning to my job. It always seemed blindingly obvious to me, but that is not the same thing as convincing someone else.

A few things got in the way as well. As part of the process the insurers require complete access to your medical records, the notes from every appointment with your GP included. When we had first been to see the GP, we had mentioned the house in France and the conversations that had happened about possibly moving there. This appeared in the notes. What did not appear in the notes was the fact that I had always intended to stay at work. As a result, this would regularly be brought up as evidence that I had intended to leave my job, so that my not returning to work was simply reflective of that decision, rather than my inability to do so.

In addition, the insurers often referred to the irregularity of my visits to the GP – if I was so ill, why was I not seeing my GP more regularly? This made no sense to me. I was seeing my psychiatrist monthly and my therapist weekly and my medication was on repeat prescription – what was the point of troubling the GP?

The process of the insurance claim was itself really damaging to my wellbeing. What if the initial claim was refused – how could we manage financially as a family? The anxiety around that was huge. Thankfully, the claim was accepted, but then came six-monthly reviews, which recreated the same initial anxiety about the outcome. The first review went fine and the claim was continued. The second time around, however, it was rejected, the confirmation coming in a short, formal letter days before Christmas 2012. I was wretched. No one could believe the decision, not me, not my psychiatrist, not the insurance broker, not any of my friends nor the HR team at work. We appealed it and complained to the ombudsman and eventually managed to extract a settlement from them many months later, but the experience set me back hugely in terms of my health.

Friday 13th October

I have been completing the form for the insurance claim. Aside from describing symptoms and all that, I had to give a weekly activity schedule. It can sound very busy, so much so that you think If he is doing all this then what's the problem? Of course, what it does not show is the huge anxiety associated with large parts of the activity.

And when I look at it, I realise just how much of the time I spend on my own. Because people scare me. I spend hours in the shed on my woodwork. I am surprised Lucy has not been suspicious of what is going on in there. I am now ankle deep in sawdust and wood-shavings, so there is no chance of anything illicit going on and, if I dropped a fag butt in there, the whole thing would go up in seconds, I am sure.

I play golf on my own. I walk the dog on my own. I go to therapy on my own – although there is a therapist there, or at least there is when I have my eyes open and I assume she is not nipping in and out when my eyes are closed – but my journey is on my own. The evenings are in the company of my family largely, and sometimes with friends, but the daytime is quite solitary, even though Lucy is here. We do our own things.

And of course, all my activity, whether singular or in a group, is a massive chasm away from the life of a professional city lawyer advising demanding and intelligent clients and managing a team of

25 lawyers. So the fact that I can manage a meal with friends or a pint at the pub does not mean that I am better.

Today we had my mother-in-law and her husband round for lunch. I had not really thought about what it would be like. I think I have only seen them once or twice since being ill. I barely said a word all meal. I was feeling very shaky and when I did try to speak I found myself taking great pauses to collect my thoughts and get the right words. Even when I do get the sentence out, no one seems remotely interested anyway. It is a while since I have felt so unwell in company. Goodness knows what they thought – if of course they noticed. But at least it might make them realise it is not all some big act and that I should (and could) just pull myself together. Anyway, it really takes it out of me.

I have promised myself a game of golf. I dither about whether to go because I feel so crap and scared and shaky, but on the other hand I have been looking forward to golf and do find it something to immerse myself in, be mindful in, focus only on the golf and nothing else, so I make myself go and end up having a nice round.

CHAPTER 21

MY BUILDING APPRENTICESHIP

Monday 31st October

Well it has been a long time hasn't it? I spent two weeks in France over half-term. I drove down with the girls for the first week then Lucy joined me with Jude the following week.

I spent the first couple of days mowing, strimming, and gathering leaves and generally getting on top of the land, which was satisfying and something you can just throw yourself at.

Then I had a chat with Dave down the road about the need for an extension to the retaining wall around the pool in order to keep in the calcaire needed to provide a bed for the paving stones, and about the whole paving project generally. [Calcaire is a local building material comprising differently graded sizes of small stones to provide a solid base – think gravel but white and slightly bigger stones.] *What I said was that I wanted him to take charge of the project but that I would like to do as much with him as I can. We talked about the wall and he said there was no magic to it, he would tell me what needed to be done, show me how to do it and I can then get on with it. I mentioned my plan for a bricklaying course at which he scoffed saying you don't need a course to do that, 'It's bloody simple is bricklaying.' I showed him my soft hands and explained how they were lawyers' hands, half the size of his, that weren't up to this sort of thing, but he was having none of it.*

So, he gave me a shopping list of materials to buy, got me round to his place to pick up tools, including his cement mixer, and then I went to the builders' merchant with the shopping list. They spoke little English. My French will extend to a number of things but, given I have no idea what I am talking about in English, building-wise, my French is far from adequate for the job.

On one occasion, I wanted to buy some railway sleepers to create a border, to supplement the ones already round the garden. Inevitably I did not know the word so began to explain, an interested crowd gathering around me all the while. Half translated, it went a bit like:

'So, you have a train, right?'

'Oui.'

'Under the train are what?'

'Les railles.'

'Great. Under les railles, going across them to support them you have what?'

'Ah, oui monsieur, les traverses.'

'Fantastic – les traverses. Makes perfect sense. Do you have any?'

'Non.'

Eventually they produced an English–French dictionary for building and gardening terms which was fantastic, and each time I returned to order more items I would begin by asking for the dictionary. And I ended up going back every other day as I thought I needed one more block or a bit more cement, always under-ordering until the point when I was running out of sand and realised I needed to order enough to make it worth them delivering it, so now we have a huge pile of sand for the local wildlife to "faire la toilette" in over the winter.

The initial list included 20 cubic metres of calcaire, 5 cubic metres of sand, a load of cement, blocks, steels, and other bits and pieces. I was told it would be three or maybe four lorry loads and I began to get a little bit nervous.

The first truckload arrived mid-afternoon. I knew it was here because I heard a loud engine noise as the driver tried to manoeuvre his vehicle backwards into our drive. I went out to greet him in my cheeriest French accent which was received with the dullest of grunts and a disdainful glance at my outstretched hand.

The load contained the bricks, cement, steels, other bits, and the sand – this being tipped out the back of the truck. He then said I had three truckloads of calcaire to come.

Now the sand was a big pile – 5 cubic metres of the stuff. That looked pretty impressive and I was far from clear I would need anything like that amount for the building I had in mind, but who was I to know – but three times that amount of calcaire was a terrifying prospect. I had worked it out on the basis that we needed to raise the level around the pool by 20cm and the whole area to be raised was about 100 square metres, but even so ...

Dave's first instruction was to dig a trench where I wanted the wall to go. Halfway through the dig the first batch of calcaire arrived and this time the driver was a little more cordial – I suspect he was laughing to himself about the idea of this English fool building a wall and dealing with the calcaire Mont Blanc heading my way. He negotiated the route round the house and reversed up to the pool edge to start tipping out the load. I had a few frantic moments as it looked like the entire amount was going to be discharged into, as opposed to around, the pool but I should have trusted him a little more. When it was all out of the truck we had a pile about a metre and a half high and in a circle about three metres across. He told me this was the first of three loads, laughed and went on his way to get the next load.

I made the trench for the foundation and then made my first batches of concrete to fill it in. There is something very satisfying about having filled a concrete mixer and having it mix your concrete that you are then going to use. There were a couple of hairy moments with it but, generally speaking, it was my friend, and made me feel like a real builder with proper tools, out on my own little building site.

Dave showed me how to lay the first brick, levelling it, making sure it was aligned right, in line with the existing wall, tying it in to that wall with giant nails, explaining the need to stagger the bricks both generally and around the corner and all that. And off I went. It was, as he had promised, surprising simple, and also very satisfying as I saw my edifice grow. And also totally absorbing. You think about nothing but the wall and the next size of block, and how much cement is left and when to make the next batch and so on. There were complications and it was not the most tidy of walls but it stood and, as Dave said, I was not building a house and no one would see the untidy joints etc. once we had filled it up with calcaire.

By now we had the full pile of calcaire and it was stupidly big. You could no longer see the pool from the house. The calcaire stones were too big to be moved by a normal rake so we bought a special rake designed for the job, and, with a combination of that to level off, and shovels and wheelbarrow to move it round, we spent hours and hours for several days getting it in the right places. It is not finished – there is still a day of levelling to do, followed by a tamping machine to flatten it, all of which needs to happen before winter but, back-breaking as it was, it was immensely satisfying. We had done a vast amount of really hard work which would have cost us a fair fortune to get someone else to do. And forever we will be able to look at it and say we did it.

And I say "we" because the kids all helped in a really good spirit and made a huge contribution to the overall effort in terms of both helping to do the hard graft as well as making it more enjoyable than toiling on my own.

Mentally I was at peace. I worked physically very hard and would then relax in the evening with too much wine and beer. Before Lucy arrived, I was anxious about the amount of drinking alone I was doing, but concluded it was not technically alone as the girls were there, even if they were not actually drinking. Once Lucy arrived we were having a couple of beers to quench the thirst after finishing work and then managing two bottles of wine and nudging into a third most evenings. That did mean sleeping was not a problem and often we would be waking up around 9.00am – a reflection of the tiredness caused by the work, and not just the amount of alcohol.

I have muscles now like I have never had before in my forearms, and my body still aches from all the lifting and barrowing. Despite wearing gloves, my hands are riddled with little cuts, although thankfully the cement and concrete which was permeating them has now dispersed.

I recall one evening looking out at the land and thinking, Yes, we have taken on a lot here, there is a lot of work just to keep it as it is, let alone make changes, but we can manage it – I am on top of it and I enjoy the challenge.

I had few, if any, moments of anxiety. I did meditate a little but generally took a break from activity schedules and all that because they just seemed not relevant, and in any event, I knew each day would be filled with hard work, and I planned from day-to-day, and sometimes a little beyond the next day, what I would be doing and generally stuck to it.

I got ratty with the kids a couple of times, not least when one hit the other with a shovel or something and caused him or her to down tools in tears, but I reckon that is kind of understandable!

I got myself quite worked up for the arrival of Lucy and Jude. We were to meet them from the airport, and I decided that we would do some food shopping on the way to the airport and also grab a burger for supper. I did not want Lucy arriving and saying we had not cleaned, or thought of what she would want, or for her to feel that she had to go shopping immediately. But I also wanted to have done as much as possible on the work front so as to be able to receive her praise for all we had achieved. So that day I was still building at 6.15 or something, then had a race to clear up for the day, shave and shower, get to the supermarket in time to shop before it closed at 7.15, then get to Bordeaux, have a burger and be at the airport to meet them in arrivals. And all the time I was adding complications – get that cleaned, let's get some cold bubbly for her which means taking a bottle chiller to the supermarket, let's get a sign to hold up at the airport etc., etc. So, I ended up stressed about it all, unnecessarily.

Even at the end I was worried about finding the way and getting a text from her to say they had landed when we were still *chomping burgers, then rushed to get there in time, only for them to take nearly an hour to get through to the arrivals hall, meaning we had a good 20-minute wait in the end. The problem was trying to do too much and not keeping things in perspective. As ever ...*

CHAPTER 22

GUY FAWKES HAS A LOT TO ANSWER FOR

One of the local schools puts on a firework display every year toraise money for the school. It is a short walk from where we lived. Many of our family friends would go and one of the families had always had everyone back for supper afterwards, kids in the front room with TV and sausages, parents in the kitchen with wine and sausages. That family had recently moved from the area and so we had volunteered to host the after-display get-together in their place.

Monday 7ᵗʰ November (Evening)

Fireworks on Saturday. Whose idea was it that I should take the kids while Lucy stayed at home cooking for the hordes that were to descend on us afterwards?

Lucy does not like fireworks at the best of times so it kind of made sense that she should stay at home but crowds ... umm. I do not like them at all at the moment. Crowds in the dark are even worse. You do not know who or what is around you, but you know there are people everywhere and you cannot escape or get away. And then you do not know where the kids are because they have all pushed through to the kids' enclosure at the front, so you are worrying about them, and then, of course, every second there is an enormous flash and a great bang. Bloody terrifying from start to finish. And slightly pointless – well more than slightly pointless from the perspective of my enjoyment and wellbeing.

It is like going on a fairground ride – the waltzer is the worst for me. You pay an exorbitant amount of cash and then get on the ride, have the bar snapped down in front of you and then the ride starts. Then you start getting spun madly around and you are scared witless, feeling sick, desperate for the ride to end, begging it to stop and begging the operator not to spin you any more – and then thinking, Hang on I have just paid decent money for this!

Well, I am there having forked out £20 or something for the tickets, then a bit more for some plastic tat stick that will glow in the dark for precisely 65 seconds until it is used by one of the kids to hit one of the others, and then fall apart ... and I see the sparks as another rocket goes off and I am thinking, Please don't bang, please, please, don't bang. I am willing myself to follow it up in the sky and prepare myself for the bang and to know it is coming and not to be afraid, but every time it makes me jump and I get closer to tears, at least I would do if the meds did not stop me from actually crying. All I get is the convulsing and the despair, without the relief of the drops down my face. Every now and then, perhaps because of the rain earlier, a rocket fails to go off and I am the one person out of the hundreds-strong crowd who is secretly rather pleased.

Like I do with the waltzer, I am willing it to end. And at last it does, but not before they have done what seemed the final set and I am relaxing and thinking of home and then they find a whole other batch of rockets which catch us all by surprise. I did not realise quite how bad it had been until it ended and then I felt myself shaking, panicking, my breathing all over the place, unable to stand without someone supporting me. Horrible, horrible, horrible. The walk back was the worst, with bangs going off at every side from people's home displays. I was a wreck when I got home.

I have nothing to do. I have kept up a fairly constant level of activity, jobs to do, visiting people, etc., but there is no DIY project here to do – the painting of the office is on hold while we work out whether we are going to sell the house or not – and I have no other great plans of how to spend my time, so the days lie ahead unfilled. I need to do something about that and so spent some time this evening making contact with my parents and with friends to try to fix up some dates.

I filled today with some shopping, dog walking, and cooking. I also started once again filling in my activity schedule because actually I did a fair bit today in the end, and spent some quality time with the kids doing homework and playing games.

In general, over the last few days I have felt low, depressed. I have been more agitated than recently, more shaky. I have been more tired as well. But I do feel more at ease with the idea of not going back to work – I guess I mean that I am more comfortable with the idea that I am ill and will continue to be so for a while at least. That is how it is and there is nothing to be done about it and nothing to be ashamed of or worried about.

CHAPTER 23

TOO MUCH OF A GOOD THING?

Saturday 3ʳᵈ December – Onboard Ferry Back to England

I have just spent a little under two weeks on my own in France. It was originally planned for 10 days but ended up being extended to get some jobs finished.

I did a lot of work. I finished levelling the calcaire and tamped it down.

Pausing there, tamping represented another big step into the world of manly construction work. Sometimes called a whacker plate, a tamping machine is basically a really heavy metal plate that, petrol driven, bounces up and down to compress and flatten the ground. The idea here was to press down and level out the calcaire in order (once it had settled over the winter) to provide a base for the patio around the pool.

You don't own whacker plates, you hire them. So, I had to go to a proper builder's merchant with all sorts of plant and machinery available for hire. I hauled the machine into the front seat of my little convertible Peugeot, the top down to accommodate the machine's handle, and drove home through the French countryside. In films, men always have their true love beside them as they drive top down in the sunshine, her hair blowing backwards in the wind. I had my whacker plate.

Using the whacker plate is like nothing I have ever experienced. Having got it in place on the calcaire, I started her up, grabbed hold of the handle and gently applied the throttle and it just took over my whole body. It is this loud and very heavy bouncing thing, pulling your arms out of their sockets as it inches forward, while at the same time sending deep vibrations through your entire body. I soon learnt to empty my bowels before a whacking session.

Back in the half-term we had bought some outside lights for the covered outdoor eating area which is becoming known as the café. An expat spark called Mario was supposed to come and fit them but never turned up. Dave down the road says electrics are easy, so I decide to give it a go.

The first job was to work out where the nearest supply was which meant venturing into an end area of attic accessed from outside and only high enough to stoop in.

My enquiries took me to a dark corner where I found an electric cable junction box with its lid hanging off. It was a mess, but at least I had a source.

Fixing the lights onto the wall where I wanted them was pretty easy and quite satisfying. You get the pleasure of seeing the lights up on the wall and there is demonstrable progress – no light yet though. Attaching wires to them was also no great challenge. The difficult part was connecting them all to the power source, via a switch. I spent hours up in that loft space, most of my tools arrayed around me, painstakingly and methodically working out what needed connecting where and slowly getting it done.

And then there is the moment of truth. I had worked for more than a day on this job, having been variously frustrated, patient, confused, angry, and much else besides, on something, electrics, which was a completely new thing for me and something that previously I would never once have thought of doing myself. I needed to turn back on the house power supply and then flick my new switch. If it worked then brilliant – success, jubilation, celebration, smugness, and satisfaction would pour out of me down the valley and probably send ripples all the way to South-West London. If nothing happened, however, then it was abject failure because I had given my all to this, had had to think really hard how to get it right and, if it did not work, then I would have no option but to give up in despair.

It was an all-or-nothing moment, so with the house power on, I flicked my switch and, for an agonising moment, nothing happened, before slowly the new, energy-efficient bulbs warmed up and one, two, three, four lights lit up around the café. It was a fantastic moment and one I enjoyed for some time flicking my switch and smiling in satisfaction. I did that – Look, lights, they work, I did that!

Aside from pruning and cleaning and various smaller repair tasks, the other big job undertaken was to redecorate the office. I had envisioned this as being a relatively simple job of filling in some holes in the walls, cleaning the walls and ceiling and then painting them all – how foolish.

One of the pieces of furniture we were left by the previous owners was a huge, ornate, free-standing cupboard / cabinet which ran along two thirds of one wall. Behind this cabinet I could see that the wall was a bit oddly shaped – it had a distinct bulge to it.

I thought about pretending I had not seen anything. Could I just push the cabinet back where it was and paint round it for example? Would anyone ever know? Who cares if they did? But something in me said, No, you need to do this properly and you need to know what is going on under there.

I summon Dave to have a look. He says get a wire brush and clear off everything that is loose. When I am done, there is a large mound of rubble all around me and a large arch shaped area in the wall, several inches deep in parts. I need to plaster the hole. Plastering is easy Dave tells me, no problem, you'll get it done in no time. So, I go round to his gaffe to collect tools and a two minute demonstration of how to mix the plaster and then apply it. Somehow, I know this is going to get messy.

After much hesitation and prevarication, I decide there is nothing for it but to get cracking and see how it goes. I find that it is not impossible to get the plaster onto the wall. The problems are getting it smooth and then knowing when to stop. After several hours I down tools. It is dark outside, I am tired, and I am not getting it any smoother by my repeated attempts to throw on another layer and really get it flat this time. The roughness will match the rest of the house and I can always put the cabinet back in place to cover the mess.

I know that the plaster will drink up paint, so, I go back to the lady at the builders' yard to say I want some cheap white paint to seal off the plaster, because, as I explain (and she ignores, much to my disappointment after my wonderful display of both language and national obsession), 'Je sais que le plâtre va boire beaucoup du peinture mais je préfère que c'est le vin de pays, pas le grand vin de Bordeaux.' – I know that the plaster will drink a lot but I would prefer it drinks plonk rather than a fine Bordeaux. She sells me some plaster-sealing paint and off I go.

The office ended up taking the best part of a week. It meant I did not get time to do the carpentry I had planned or some other bits and pieces, but it was a challenge and I took it on and learnt some new things and the result is not that bad.

So, there was a lot of work, but it was as much my obsession about it all that stopped me taking time to do other, purely relaxing, things. I had a list of jobs with a rough idea of how long each would take, and I was constantly working out what was next, how many things I could be getting on with, always working.

Even the final morning was mad. I finished the painting in the office, then put the furniture back and a rug down, finished clearing up my painting equipment, swept and mopped the kitchen, toilet and hall, (after having my breakfast), hung out some washing, took the rubbish and recycling to the bins and the glass to the bottle bank and various other little things. That was all before leaving at 9.45, after a shower.

I was obsessed about getting it all done – it all has to be just so – I am unable to say 'Oh fuck it, it does not matter.' I do not want Lucy coming and thinking, Well he could have done this or that.

And I do not want myself thinking I have not done as much as I can do. My head is full of voices judging me, demanding perfection of me. I pretend they are other people, but it is really just me. And in the process, I drive myself to the limit and that is the reason I am in this mess in the first place.

That was the last entry I wrote in my diary. What follows, therefore, is from my recollection a few years on. I have no idea why I did not carry on writing. I don't think it was a conscious decision. I suspect that in the build-up to Christmas that year I was busy and found less time to write and, like all things, once you get out of the habit, it is hard to get back into it. The longer you leave it, the less likely it is that you will start again.

It is an informative point to have stopped at though. I recognise and recall only too well the obsessive working, urging myself on and on with feelings of obligation – I have to do this, I have to get it right. Where is the voice from the Priory telling me, 'Enough'? It seems that even though I may have learnt many new skills, building, plastering, electrics and more, I had yet to learn new ways of thinking, to give myself a break, to allow myself to rest and to fail. My best mate Mike recalls a regular incident from our early years working together as trainee solicitors. It would get to 6.00pm or so and he would decide that it was time for a pint in the local pub. He would stick his head round my door and ask if I fancied joining him and I would always have just one more thing I needed to get finished. I could never just stop and say, 'Yep, that'll do for a day's work.'

There was some guilt involved, I think. I felt I needed to justify the time I had taken away from the kids and Lucy. I wanted to be able to show them that I was not sitting back enjoying myself, but really making an effort. I very much doubt the kids gave any thought to it at all of course. There was also a developing sense of the amount of time I was taking away from work and wanting to be able to say (to myself, I think, but perhaps to others) that although I was not yet well enough to go back to my old work, I did use the time effectively. Somehow, I could not accept that just getting myself better was sufficient use of my time.

Of course, being active physically is good for your wellbeing and recovery. Similarly, learning new skills is helpful, as is having a sense of purpose. It also meant that Lucy and I were not tripping over each other the whole time at home.

CHAPTER 24

REPORT FROM THE FRONT

That December, conscious that I had not been in contact with lots of people for many months, who may or may not have heard rumours of my being ill, with Lucy's help I sent a round-robin email to family and friends to give them an update.

Dear all,

Apologies for the general email but thought I would send an update on what is happening to me to answer lots of questions and worries people may or may not have. Some of you will know some of this already so apologies for boring you.

I am still on a high dose of medication to keep the anxiety in check and it generally works, although when I get tired I tend to get a bit jumpy.

I am seeing my consultant less regularly – once every month or so. He is happy with my progress. As he says, there will be good days and bad days, ups and downs, but as long as the general trend is upwards then that is good. I know that I am feeling much better than six, or even two, months ago and am capable of much more than I was in the summer. He reminds me that I was in emergency treatment in hospital only a few months ago so I must not be impatient with progress. I have weekly cognitive behavioural therapy treatment (CBT) which is helping and will continue for some time. It looks at the core beliefs that I have developed over the years from all the experiences I have had, about my relationship with the world and the people in it, and which then affect how I behave. For those beliefs that are unhelpful to me it seeks to challenge them and replace them with more helpful beliefs and behaviours.

And the medics tell me that those core beliefs kind of lie at the heart of my problems. I was doing a highly stressful job but no more stressful than lots of other people do and no doubt a good deal less stressful than some. They say that my problem was in the way that I dealt with that stress and the day-to-day demands of life. My response, created by my core beliefs, produced an unhelpful reaction which compounded the stress rather than relieving it.

Some people have seen me recently and said, 'He seems alright, why is he still at home? When is he going to go back to work, what are his plans etc.?' And I can understand that. Compared to several months ago I am much improved and can sit round a table and chat and behave in normal ways. It does tire me out and there are days when I can't even do this, but that is not the point. There is an enormous gap between being able to do little things once a day on the one hand, and on the other dealing with the unrelenting stress of the job I was doing.

Imagine a football player in the premier league. The demands of playing premier league football place huge demands and stresses on the physical body of the player. He gets injured. He will have some hospital treatment and then undergo rehab treatment. The doctors may be able to say that they expect him to be able to get back to where he was in due course, and may be able to say that they would normally expect it to be in, say, six-to-twelve months, or some kind of time frame. But it is a long road and there is no guarantee that he will ever be able to get back to that level. He may be able to go for a walk in the park, may be able to go running, may be *able to kick a ball about with his mates and maybe even play for the reserve team. But all of that is a long way short of the demands of a premier league game.*

In the demands it makes of me mentally, my job feels a little like the physical demands of a top footballer. So right now, I may have made enough progress to be able to deal with day-to-day stuff – but that is a long way short of being able to deal with the stress of the job.

Just like the footballer, there is nothing I would like more than to be well enough to perform at the highest level. I am not shirking anything or shying away from anything. That is not my way. If I felt even half well enough to get back to work, I would be champing at the bit and having to be restrained.

I hope that makes some sense.

Encouraged by my psychiatrist I am looking to build into my routine some more social contact. I have been helping out with some maintenance stuff at the school opposite where Jude still goes. Painting, clearing brambles, cleaning graffiti, the kind of jobs that the caretaker never finds time for. Most of it is probably Jude's mess anyway so it kind of seems fair.

I have been doing various DIY jobs around the house and also on our French house. As well as new skills, it is rewarding and empowering to be able to achieve things, and to do things that we would previously have paid people to do. Of course, we may find in due course that we need to pay someone to clear up the mess I have made, but for the moment the lights come on when you flick the switch, and the plaster (or at least most of it) remains stuck to the wall.

Until now I have been receiving sick pay from my work. That has now run out, but I have had my application for permanent health insurance accepted. This will mean that the insurers replace a good part (but not all) of my previous income, so that is reassuring – we can afford to live and also a third party, the insurer, for whom this is going to cost a deal of cash, agrees that I am too unwell to go back to my job. So I am not imagining all of this or making it up.

Lucy continues to be an angel to me. She no longer needs to lead me by the elbow to wherever we are going and whisper in my ear about what is going on but does still have to shoulder much more than her fair share of the burden of keeping the Martins afloat and does so without the limited support she ever received from a properly functioning me, and she keeps an eye out for me and what I am up to and how I am coping. At the same time, she has finished another book, and has developed a new business tutoring kids and adults in French, Spanish, and English, in groups and individually.

The kids are wonderful, too, and aside from the usual winter colds everyone is well. They are all doing well with school and music and sports and all sorts and make us proud every day.

Happy Christmas to all if we are not going to see you and thanks for your ongoing concern and support – especially all that you give and have given to Lucy.

Richard x

CHAPTER 25

EXILE IN FRANCE

We muddled onwards to Christmas, deciding to spend Christmas itself in France. Relations between Lucy and me were strained already. That Christmas in France tested them to their limits and was not, in hindsight, the best idea. I think few of us would say we enjoyed that festive period as a family.

In January, I attended a week's carpentry course at a building skills training centre in Dartford. I had wanted to learn some new skills to use in France and had decided carpentry would be the most useful – I did not feel I could justify the time and financial cost of staying on for more than a week and learning other skills. Some of the other people on the course were, however, going for the full immersion, spending many weeks progressing through plumbing, electrics, brickwork, plastering, tiling, carpentry, and more.

There was also a test involved for me – would I be able to deal with the anxiety of being around different people, in a different and strange place with the noise of a workshop going on the whole time in the background? Although I wanted to try, there was a huge level of anxiety attached to it, so it was a relief to meet the class on the first day and not feel the need to run to my car and escape. Interestingly, we did introductions around the group, including why we were on the course. Most of the class were tradesmen looking to extend their skills. A city law firm partner off work sick with mental health problems and using the course, in part, as therapy, therefore, stuck out a bit, but I was accepted readily enough, and with kindness.

It was a really great experience. There is the learning of new skills, the mindfulness of focusing on your work in hand – the joint you are chiselling out for example, or the door you are learning to hang – and the sense of achievement, of progress.

Meanwhile, back at home, tension between Lucy and me continued. I was still on a relatively high dose of medication at this point, while still experiencing regular occasions of acute anxiety in the house. This created tension for Lucy and the kids as they watched me dissolve into tears and shaking at the sound of a plate dropping or a door slamming. Lucy was also looking to the future and wanting to know where she and I stood as a couple. She wanted to know how I felt about her and whether I wanted us to stay together. The truth was I did not know. The medication, in taking the edge off the extremes of anxiety and depression, was numbing my emotions more generally. I did not know what I felt. So I could not give Lucy an honest answer, other than 'I don't know', which of course was not that encouraging from her perspective.

I think also there may have been something else at play. I have talked about how I had in many respects not learnt to make choices for myself, doing what it seemed others wanted me to do, or what duty seemed to dictate. Here I was, being presented with one of the biggest choices in my life: in effect, did I want to stay with my wife and the mother of my children? I did not really understand how it had come to that. I did not know how to make a decision and I knew it was one that I alone could make. The medication certainly clouded my thoughts, but I suspect there was a paralysis of choice there too, not knowing how to make a decision.

And so, after much discussion with my psychiatrist and therapist, we agreed that I would go and live in France on my own for an extended period of several months. The purpose was to stop bothering the family with my anxiety, to let me spend time somewhere that seemed to make me happy and fulfilled, and for me slowly to come off my medication in a controlled way, so as to be able to re-connect with my emotions and be able to talk to Lucy on an emotional level.

Allied to that, and part of the process of recovery, was to give myself a purpose day-to-day. I was going to have the time to work on the house in France in an ordered, planned way, rather than cramming projects into short visits. I would also learn to take responsibility for, and control over, my existence, and to strive for what I wanted to do and achieve – to plan my days and weeks around what I felt I needed to be doing, rather than around other people and their needs and desires.

Gradually over the previous months, I had started playing more of a role in the family home in London, looking after the children in particular. But that was the role Lucy had always fulfilled and with the kids at the age they were, there was just not enough there to require the two of us. I was therefore taking away some of her role and purpose, and going away to France allowed her to take that back. At the same time, my own sense of wellbeing was becoming too bound up with how Lucy was feeling. I felt like I was responsible for how she felt. As I sailed off from Portsmouth one night in late February / early March, drinking a beer as I watched the ship slowly pull away and leave England behind, I felt a sense of relief and release. I did not have to worry about all of that for a while.

I ended up staying in France until the May half-term holiday I think. They were at once both challenging and gentle times. I had a simple routine. I would work on house and garden projects during the day, then spend the evenings watching box sets of DVDs brought from England.

I also spent many hours on a fiendish jigsaw that Lucy's mother had given me. I was doing it on a table in the lounge and it was always sitting there whenever I wandered in, reminding me of its incomplete state. Because it was so difficult, it gave very little joy, and, the progress being so slow, very little satisfaction. But I felt duty bound to continue with it, and so I did for months until, on the spur of a moment, I decided I had had enough of being controlled by it. Breaking up the work I had done and putting it back in the box felt too sad, that I was wasting all the time and effort which would only have to be repeated as and when it came out again. The only way to stop that happening was to destroy it, and so I took huge (but guilty) delight one evening in throwing the entire thing on the fire and watching it blaze away. Perhaps that jigsaw was a metaphor for how I felt, broken into too many pieces and not yet ready or able to find a way of putting them back together again.

There were various house and garden projects – not all of them would have been in this period but the passage of time has blurred the memory of what and when.

I cleared the old vegetable garden and replanted it and we ended up with lots of carrots and potatoes, some beans, and courgettes which carried on well into the autumn. I was there when the cherries ripened in May and experienced the joy of delicious, ripe, sweet, juicy cherries hanging in their armfuls on the tree waiting for me to enjoy them. Picking them resulted in cherry juice running down my arms. I ate huge quantities, gave away more, made many jars of jam to keep and to give away and pickled a whole lot more in different jars of cognac, gin and vodka – delights that I am still enjoying years later.

The damson tree also fruited that year, resulting in damson cakes and jam. An old peach tree, long since on its last gnarled legs, coughed up a few choice treats and then later in the year we were buried in figs from the trees that surround the house.

We also planted some new trees to replace those that were dying off. Meanwhile, the old cherry tree has played its part, spawning a number of young trees growing in its protective shade, so they can be planted out in due course. It feels part of an ongoing cycle of renewal and nurture, even if I may not be around to appreciate the fruits of the labour.

I decided to demolish the rickety and ineffective barbecue stand and replaced it with a stone shed built next to the bread oven whose roof I then replaced and extended to cover the new shed too. I also then renovated the bread oven, which we have since used for various pizza evenings.

Having renovated what was there, I started to get ambitious and set about designing a roof structure that would form a pitch with the sloped roof off the bread oven and a covered eating / play area underneath. It was a lot of work – even the base needed 15 or so tons of concrete to be mixed and spread. I did the vast majority of it myself, only calling for help when some particularly long and thick timbers needed hoisting onto pillars at a height of some 10 feet or so.

One of the most satisfying moments came later in the summer when I was still working as the sun was beginning to set. I was standing on top of the nearly finished roof, sawing and nailing timbers into place. I was wearing just some scraggy shorts and some boots, my back was aching with the effort of another day's hard labour, saw in one hand, hammer in the other, sun still warm on my back as I stretched it out. I felt like a man. I felt fulfilled. I felt proud of what I had done. I felt happy and at one with where I was and who I was.

When I sit under that roof now I cannot quite believe the sheer balls I must have had to think I could just get on and do it. The first few visits to the house after it was complete always involved a slight degree of nervousness around whether it would still be standing. I will not claim it is the most perfectly finished construction job in the world, but it's the most perfectly finished one I have ever undertaken (and completed) and I reckon it will last me out and, probably, my grandchildren, too.

When the weather was warmer and I could open up the pool, I could treat myself at the end of the day with a plunge into the cooling waters.

But it was far from always blissful. Every job involved multiple setbacks and complications. And the list of tasks to be done seldom seemed to shorten – although that was double-edged in the sense that I had a constant sense of purpose and had no worries about what I would do when the current work was done, because it plainly never would be.

And I had to make every decision myself, not just about the work to be done, what, how, when, but simple things like what to eat, when to wash clothes, bedding etc. I was not relaxing but in a constant fervour of activity, consumed by the rhythm of hard work – not legal work now but hard labour.

In my constant drive to keep working, to take on ever more difficult and laborious tasks, I was hurting myself. I was not looking after myself, self-flagellating in a sense. And because there was no one there to tell me to stop, I carried on, working well into the evenings on a regular basis when the weather allowed.

If the hard work was intended to keep anxiety and depression at bay, it was not always successful. Although I had stopped writing my diary, I did from time to time try to capture my thoughts and feelings in poetry. It's not going to win any prizes, but for me was an effective way to capture my feelings.

The solitude too was double-edged. I did not have to worry about Lucy's state of mind, nor risk being driven to anxiety by the kids' noise or fighting or questions. I could control my own time and was, on one level at least, answerable only to myself. The kids did visit, and I would talk to them from time to time on the phone or Skype. It was never quite satisfying, always feeling like a set piece with too many layers of expectation when all we really wanted was just to hug and lounge about together. And I could see Dave and Cher down the road and did get to know other neighbours and took part in some of the local social events. I would also be too chatty with people in shops, largely to enjoy a bit of company and take comfort in hearing their voices and mine. But very often I would spend days on my own. Mealtimes brought it home in particular.

At one stage, I had heard mewing for several days and a scuffling when I went to investigate its source. I was on the roof one day when I heard the mewing again and then a splash – a kitten had fallen down the well.

Using the swimming pool net on its longest extension, I just managed to get down to the water level in the well and scoop the sodden mess up out of the dark waters. As I gently lifted her out she took fright and jumped back down the well again. On the second attempt I got her out and found her some milk and tuna to feast on. She was tiny and there was no sign of mum anywhere. She would cower from me, suggesting she had had very little contact with humans and would not let me within a couple of metres. I wandered round to our nearest neighbours to ask if they were missing a kitten. The answer was that they had a stray cat that lived in their barn which had probably had kittens and the next time mine fell into the well I should leave it there. The kindness of the French does not always extend to their animals.

I fed my new friend for a few days, but she stopped appearing. Maybe she caught up with mum or found a new friend or a different end, but for that short period I had had another life to support, a little test of my humanity and ability to care for others perhaps.

Ivy was, and remains, a constant and insidious menace. Its underground tentacles seem to be beneath every tree and it attempts to climb every building. The older walls of the barn were crumbling in places and when I removed the ivy to get to the stone work I could see that the ivy was actually growing within the mud bricks and stone wall. Whenever I had a spare minute to stop and stare I would notice another tree under attack and then lose my reverie as I set to work, stripping the murderous smothering tide of green from the trunk and branches, and trying to get as much out from underground as I could.

It became a metaphor for my battle with anxiety and depression – spreading itself far and wide, ready to appear anywhere at a moment's notice, to rise and smother and consume, sucking the life out of whatever supported it. At the front of the property is an old tree that has long since died but whose corpse supports a mass of ivy. The old tree is rotten within, the ivy now mostly supporting itself, aping the shape of the old beast. Every now and then a branch of ivy becomes too much for the rotten wood beneath and the monster loses another limb but still it stands, a parody of life.

That sense of being consumed by depression and anxiety, of it sucking the life from me, of the dark leaves and branches slowly entrapping me (unless I worked hard to keep them at bay) was a regular menace. There were days when I would spend the whole day going from place to place tearing out ivy, creating huge piles of the stuff which I would carry triumphantly overhead on a pitchfork to toss onto the ever-growing compost heap.

Human Touch

The hard work was taking its toll on me physically. My legs and arms were constantly tired and my back was aching. The spa a few kilometres from the house offers massage. I had been thinking about it for a while but somehow did not think I deserved it, it felt too decadent to spend time and money on myself in that way, particularly when there was work to be done.

Eventually I persuaded myself that maybe just once might be forgivable, and so I met Sophie, and from her enjoyed a number of massages over the following months, both at the spa and at her own treatment room elsewhere. I was blown away. In part it was the care and attention that another human being was paying to me and to my body, care that I had not known for some time and which I certainly did not give myself. There was also the fact of human touch. And, of course, there was the soothing effect of massage on aching muscles. But there was something much more than this and far more powerful. Every now and then, and normally at least once in each session, there would be an extraordinary feeling that all of the anxiety in my body and mind was drawn out of me through her hands. I could feel a sensation of heat coursing through my body to the point where her hands were touching me and flowing out of me through those hands. And I was left completely at peace for a while.

The second or third time this happened, I summoned my best French to try to explain this phenomenon to Sophie. I had already told her about my depression and anxiety. She finished my sentence for me because, she said, she felt it too. She had no idea how it was happening and it was not something she had ever encountered in her work before, but she was feeling the drawing of anxiety out of me just as strongly as I was. It was the most effective means I had, and have since, found to relieve my anxiety in the short-term and I would visit her fortnightly when I could.

A New Man?

My daily work before I was ill was based around the use of my brain. I had enjoyed a bit of carpentry, gardening, and the odd more challenging DIY project, but this was always a sideshow – the working self I displayed to the world, the identity I created for myself, was cerebral. This was what defined me and what provided for my family. Although I had some sense of physical self, of the rest of my body, it was largely something to move my head around from place to place.

With my brain not functioning as it had as a result of the depression and anxiety, it was as if I took on a new identity, a new self. I was learning to work with my hands, my body, alongside, or even in place of, my brain. With it, I developed a confidence in my physical self that I had hitherto not had. Clearly, I was taking on projects that I would never normally have done, and when faced with something that needed doing, my first thought began to be how I would tackle it rather than which professional I would need to engage to do it.

I also became more earthy if that makes sense, more in tune with, and absorbed by, my physical surroundings, the weather, and the turning of the seasons. I began to feel almost part of the land. Thinking in terms of Maslow's hierarchy of needs, wherever my focus had been previously, now I was tending to the basic needs of shelter and food. That felt very grounded. It felt like I was rebuilding from the bottom up, as if my hierarchy had all been called into question, or even destroyed, and I was starting again. There was also some comfort in the somewhat catastrophic notion that if the worst came to the worst and the family was left with nothing, I could care for their most basic needs – my ability to fund someone else to do so might have gone but now I could do it myself.

Coming Off the Meds

Over those months in France in the first half of 2012, I gradually reduced the dosage of my medication as agreed with my psychiatrist until I stopped taking anything at all. It seemed to go relatively easily, without any major upsurge of anxiety or depression as I lowered the dose. Looking back, I can see that I had deliberately chosen a safe place to go through this process, where the anxieties of "real life" were not ever-present, which did enable me to make the break, but was not really testing my ability to cope drug-free in that real life.

But, I managed it and was able to come back to England in the early summer, drug-free as had been the plan.

CHAPTER 26

VENTURING OUT

The rest of that summer was spent between England and France. In England, encouraged by my psychiatrist, I took on some voluntary work in a local charity shop. There were various reasons for this. It would give me a sense of purpose and existence outside of the house. It would give me some routine and limited responsibility – I would have to be there when my shift pattern required it at the very least. It would also involve interacting with other people and the public, with all of the uncertainty and scope for anxiety that entailed.

It felt like quite a big deal, but I soon settled in and got to know the other people who worked there, as well as the routine of shop work. I had had retail holiday jobs years earlier, and, as a result there was something familiar with the work, and I was pleased to be able to cope with it and be of use.

There was also another hark back to the past. The shop was a branch of FARA which raises money for Romanian orphanages. Between university and law school I had spent the best part of a year working in Bucharest on a project rehousing street children, setting up houses for them to live in, and getting them re-established in the school system and other aspects of life. It was nice to feel a re-connection with the past. FARA means "without" in Romanian. The charity exists to provide for those without in Romania, but in a strange way was also providing for me, without in a different way in London.

It was a simple but very important step, giving me the confidence to build from there. Although I knew that I had, for a while, been better than when at my lowest points, I had had a very limited level of engagement with the world. I had spent long periods on my own in France. In England I was very firmly based at, and spent much of my time in, the family home, with contact with other people quite limited and controlled. This was venturing out.

In the autumn, I took another step. I decided I wanted to test my brain and to learn something new, and enrolled on an introductory course in psychotherapy and counselling. It was a short course – perhaps one morning a week for 10 weeks or something – but was a challenge on various levels. First of all, it was in Central London, which meant committing to regular interactions with public transport and the terrors that trains and Tubes still held for me. Prior to the day of enrolment and interview for the course, I practised the journey from door to door to give myself some level of familiarity and comfort before having to do it "live", so to speak. Secondly, it would involve a group of new people, which was scary. And thirdly, it was challenging my brain, and learning something totally new, albeit at a basic level. It would require focus and concentration, things that had been in short supply on anything other than manual tasks, and golf, since I had been ill.

The choice of subject matter is perhaps obvious. I had become very interested in therapy while in the Priory, and had seen counsellors off and on ever since. The thought of returning to work in a law firm still seemed impossible to contemplate – I could not imagine ever feeling well enough to do that. So, I was wondering whether this might be an alternative career path.

The course was interesting enough. Over the weeks the anxiety of the journey, and of being in a room with others, reduced to levels with which I could cope. I would not say it was easy, by any means, but I managed and I completed the course. Encouraged by that and by my growing interest in the subject matter, I decided to apply for a foundation course in psychotherapy and counselling at a London university, now occupying the same buildings that had once housed my mother's university college many years earlier.

This was a proper, grown-up course in a real university. It ran from January to April 2013. Classes were every Saturday and Sunday through that period, with at least a day of homework to complete in between. The subject matter was complex and I was now expected to read and understand it, and then be able to discuss it at a far deeper level. It was like going back to university, which sounds silly; it wasn't *like* that, it *was* that. I got a student card, bought lots of new stationery, and got myself organised.

The classes were a mix of theory – starting with Freud and covering many of the key figures, events and themes in the history of psychotherapy – and practice. We would role play counselling with each other in triads – one person playing the role of client, one the counsellor, and one observing and feeding back to the counsellor what they had observed, good and bad.

These practical sessions were very tightly controlled at the outset. In order to create a realistic setting for the counsellor to develop her / his skills, the client was encouraged to speak about real issues affecting them. At the same time, one had to be careful about one's own welfare and not to stray into areas that might prove too challenging, for client or counsellor.

The skills were built up very gradually. At the outset, the mock sessions were short – perhaps five or ten minutes in length, and the counsellor was required simply to sit and listen, adopting a still pose that demonstrated openness, attention, and empathy, while not responding in any way to what was said. We learnt simply to listen, and of the power and gift of silence. Gradually we added in non-verbal cues, nods, facial expressions, encouraging noises, and then words, but in a controlled way. As the mock sessions got longer, we could reflect back words that the client had used and then add a question around them – 'You mentioned that you felt [x], tell me more about that.'

Gradually we built up the ability to make more perceptive observations, perhaps referencing the body language of the client, how it told the same or a different story to the words being used, or perhaps linking different aspects of what we had been told – 'You began by telling me about [y], and now you are talking about [z] and I wonder whether there is a link between the two for you?' We were always reminded to tread warily. We were not trained, experienced therapists, and we were not trying to counsel the client, but practise our skills as trainee counsellors. The focus, therefore, in terms of feedback on the session was always about what the counsellor was doing rather than the narrative from the client.

Initially the mock sessions would be conducted in chairs. Later we also used a couch where the client would be encouraged simply to speak about whatever came into her / his head, "free associating" as it is sometimes called.

Throughout it all the biggest thing we learnt, and perhaps the most challenging for people who, like me, had spent a career doling out advice, was to listen non-judgementally and to try to clear our heads of any opinions, prejudices, assumptions, advice, and expectations that we might have. These are our own, they are about us. In most kinds of therapy, it is about the client. As a result, the therapist's views, opinions and all the rest are not just completely irrelevant, but they are destructive of the therapeutic relationship, where the focus remains on the client's thoughts and feelings. The role of the counsellor is to create the safe frame in which the client can speak.

The learning experience was fantastic: hugely informative, challenging, and motivating, but something else was happening too. As a group of students, we were talking to each other in these sessions on a level and in a way that just does not happen in normal life. It was as if we existed in that environment in a pure, almost Eden-like, state. The barriers we create to maintain our distance from each other were removed and we stared into each other's souls. And of course, when you open your soul or mind to let others see in, you also allow yourself to see the stuff that is hidden away in there – those weekends were like extended therapy sessions in many ways.

Most of the time it felt safe – it could not have functioned unless the course leaders made it so. There were moments of discomfort though. Some came from the work we were doing and the challenges that entailed. Some from each other and from ourselves. On one occasion when we were together as a large group, I remember listening to another group member talking at great length, and feeling that what she was saying was wrong, and also wasteful of our time together. Because of that, it almost felt abusive of the rest of us. Rather than anger, what I experienced was a growing sense of anxiety which began to develop into panic, such that I was on the point of having to leave the room, before someone intervened to stop the person talking.

On another occasion, I was challenged about my own behaviour. At the end of each day we would spend an hour or so in small groups reflecting on the day, how we felt, etc. The agenda was fairly loose save that we had to be respectful of each other and we were not to talk about theory, but about how we were, individually and as a group. We were assigned to groups for these sessions at the outset of the course, with one of the course leaders in each group, and we remained in those groups for the entire time. In my group, the course leader was fairly silent and, while giving little guidance on what we should be talking about in the sessions, would intervene every now and then to say that what we *were* talking about was not appropriate subject matter for the session. This became increasingly frustrating for me – and I supposed for the rest of the group – that we were told what we could not discuss but given little guidance about what we could do.

After one session where a line of discussion had been abruptly cut off by one such intervention from the course leader, and after he had left the room and the rest of us were packing up our bags, I made known my frustration and (at least I think) others concurred.

At the next session, one of the group who I had got to know and like and trust began by saying that she wanted to raise something that happened at the end of the previous session and recounted what I had said. Her reason for doing so was the way in which I had violated a group dynamic. The sessions were about us as a group and any discussion about what was happening in that group should happen with the whole group, whereas I had instigated a conversation with everyone bar one person. My immediate reactions included shame at being called out in public in this way, anger at feeling betrayed by my friend, confusion about what was happening and what I had done wrong – and fear as to the repercussions.

But, of course, this was a safe learning environment so there was no reason to be afraid. We just talked about it and then I reflected on it and came to see all sorts of patterns. I had, in my mind, made the course leader into a scary person who was in control and could punish me. He was nothing of the kind. In my frustration at what I saw as the contrast between his interventions and his unwillingness to give guidance as to what we should be talking about, as opposed to simply telling us what we should not be talking about, I was acting out a frustration from my childhood. It was a feeling that there were lots of rules about how not to be, or how one should not behave, but little in the sense of positive role modelling or guidance. This was an example of transference, a therapeutic term describing how we sometimes transfer on to a current situation feelings and thoughts about a previous situation.

Also, I reflected on why I was not angry with the person who had "dobbed me in". In a funny way I was grateful to her for doing it, which seemed to reflect a desire for someone to provide order and guidance in a confusing and sometimes frightening environment.

To complete the course, we had to write a couple of essays, one a self-reflection on the development of our own self-awareness through the course, the other a more academic essay on an area of theory we had studied. I was strangely nervous about the latter, having not written an academic essay for 20 years while most of the others in the group had left study much more recently.

I had good reason to be nervous. Although my essay was passed by my tutor, and he did say that he enjoyed reading what I had written, he politely pointed out that an academic essay was intended to be more an analysis of the work of others in the field than a statement of my own personal views. Having spent 20 years being paid to provide opinions on things, and being repeatedly told not to bore clients with lengthy statements of what the law says, but rather focus on my advice as to what they should do, it was strange to be told he was, in effect, looking for the exact opposite.

The course was, on pretty much every level, a fantastic and worthwhile experience. I had had to pay for it myself – several thousand pounds from memory – which created considerable guilt / pressure to ensure that I applied myself to it and benefitted from it. But the investment was well worth it. When everyone else in the world was relaxing on their weekend, I and my bunch of fellow students would be up early making our way across wintry London to gather in a near-deserted college to study and explore ourselves. It was like we were entering into our own little world, cut off from the rest of London, cocooned for the weekend.

There was academic stimulation in abundance, but much more than that was the kindness, openness, inquisitiveness, support, and understanding of the group. I learnt much about myself and the way I interact with other people. I also got a good chunk of self-confidence back – that I could commit to and complete something, that I could manage the journeys and the anxiety of new people, that I could learn new ways of thinking and being, and that people warmed to and respected me, and were genuinely interested in me.

It opened my eyes to new ways of being with, and connecting with, people, allowing myself to be far more open with them about me and what was happening to me and how I felt. I began to answer honestly the "how are you" question. It also taught me a whole different way of helping people. I was used to people telling me their situation so I could, with the benefit of my legal knowledge and experience, advise them as to what to do and then help them to do it. Here, I learnt a whole different level of listening, where listening and making it clear that you have listened, with a bit of empathy, is often all that is needed. It was bringing and applying myself rather than my legal expertise – connecting on a very human level as opposed to the transactional level of legal advice.

I learnt the privilege of people sharing with me their most intimate concerns, fears, hopes, motivations, of the extraordinary opportunity and connection that opens up when that happens. I also learnt that it is okay for me to talk about "my stuff" and to do so in a jumbled, messed up way, without having to try to organise and package it. Just putting it all out there on the table. Just by doing so you get to see for yourself, hear for yourself, what is really going on inside you, and you learn to accept it for what it is, as it is, without having to apologise for it, disguise or excuse it, or make any sense of it. But once it is out there, you can then pick through it if you want, and the other person can help, too, if you both want. You won't get anywhere, however, without knowing what is there, acknowledging it for what it is and accepting it, owning it.

Part of what enabled me to be so open, to explore the deepest parts of my thoughts and feelings without censoring what I was saying, was the realisation that I was not being judged. I have always feared that people are constantly sitting in judgement on me, ready to condemn me for my actions, thoughts, or feelings; and so I learnt to keep them hidden, or at the very least to pass them through a fine filter before deciding whether to expose them.

I had developed a way of speaking that was careful and deliberate, pausing to make sure that the sentences were carefully and correctly formulated to convey exactly the message I thought appropriate. Part of this is just legal training. Lawyers deal in words and fight their battles based on the words used by others and so you learn to pick yours carefully. But part was also this fear of judgement. Whose judgement was I fearing? In my early years, it had no doubt been an external judge – parents, brothers, God. In later life I feared, often no doubt incorrectly, Lucy's judgement. I am sure, however, that I had long since learnt to sit in judgement on myself.

This came to me following one end-of-day group session when one of the group talked about their experiences of miscarriage. This called to mind the miscarriage that Lucy and I had experienced before we were married. The pregnancy had been the catalyst for our getting engaged and making wedding plans and then the pregnancy ended suddenly one morning. I talked about this in the group and about how at the time some people had responded with a bit of 'Well perhaps it was for the best,' a reaction that I railed against in the group.

Leaving the session, I had a strange sense of not having been honest, not having told the whole truth. As I reflected on this overnight I realised what I had long suppressed – that in the flood of emotions that morning so many years ago, one of the different feelings I had had was one of relief. It was not the primary reaction. There was grief and there was concern and love for Lucy and much else, and it was these that I acted upon. But there was relief too – perhaps it had been for the best in some way. Because I found that thought, that feeling, to be ugly, wrong, uncaring, I had suppressed it – at the time and ever since, and again in the group session.

With much trepidation, I decided to raise this in the session the following day, fearful of the judgement of my fellow group members, but eager at the same time to take a risk, to explore what this would be like. To my surprise, there was no judgement from the group, but rather a supportive understanding and appreciation of my honesty, and that helped me in accepting the feelings that I had had. I had long heard and used the mantra that there are not good and bad feelings but simply feelings – they are what they are, it is what you do with them that may be good or bad. Here was an example of me applying that to myself and allowing myself to have feelings of that kind, forgiving myself in some way. But it was also more than forgiveness – for that implies a wrong that requires forgiveness – it was more a sense of acceptance.

The openness, support, and understanding we showed to each other as a group took time to develop over the months of the course. A big deal was rightly made of the ending of the course, and the final day was a series of different exercises and events to mark that ending. We were each invited to bring something that had meaning to us and which spoke to us of our experiences on the course, and which we could share with the group.

I chose the poem, 'The Journey of the Magi' by T. S. Eliot. Eliot describes the journeys the wise men undertook to visit and pay homage to the infant Jesus, their struggles with snow, hostile environments, recalcitrant camels, and more besides, as well as the transformation that they experienced. This left them feeling at odds with their old worlds, their old ways of being. In choosing the poem I had in mind the physical journeys we had each made to attend the course – there had been snow in the early weeks and at various times our camels, the Tube or trains, had not operated, whether through strike action or planned repair work. On another level, though, there was the spiritual journey we had each been on, developing a new level of understanding of ourselves and of each other, an understanding which felt at odds with much of the culture and ways of being in the "real world", outside the confines of our course and group.

That sense of journey was also reflected in a poem another group member shared, 'Ithaka', written by C.P. Cavafy in 1911:

As you set out for Ithaka
hope the voyage is a long one,
full of adventure, full of discovery.
Laistrygonians and Cyclops,
angry Poseidon–don't be afraid of them:
you'll never find things like that on your way
as long as you keep your thoughts raised high,
as long as a rare excitement
stirs your spirit and your body.
Laistrygonians and Cyclops,
wild Poseidon–you won't encounter them
unless you bring them along inside your soul,
unless your soul sets them up in front of you.

Hope the voyage is a long one.
May there be many a summer morning when,
with what pleasure, what joy,
you come into harbours seen for the first time;
may you stop at Phoenician trading stations
to buy fine things,
mother of pearl and coral, amber and ebony,
sensual perfume of every kind–
as many sensual perfumes as you can;
and may you visit many Egyptian cities
to gather stores of knowledge from their scholars.

Keep Ithaka always in your mind.
Arriving there is what you are destined for.
But do not hurry the journey at all.
Better if it lasts for years,
so you are old by the time you reach the island,
wealthy with all you have gained on the way,
not expecting Ithaka to make you rich.

Ithaka gave you the marvellous journey.
Without her you would not have set out.
She has nothing left to give you now.

And if you find her poor, Ithaka won't have fooled you.
Wise as you will have become, so full of experience,
you will have understood by then what these Ithakas mean.[2]

That poem now adorns the wall above my desk at home, reminding me of the importance of now, of the journey, rather than whatever destination we may or may not attain.

Shortly after the course ended I was in one of those shops that sells cute things for your house, whitewashed wooden decorations, cushions and signs with maxims for how to live your life. I tend to be pretty sceptical (indeed, dismissive would be a fairer description) of the signs, but one took my eye and now hangs in my flat and is deliberately in my line of sight countless times a day: "Life is not about waiting for the storm to pass. It is about learning to dance in the rain." I know that I did, and to some extent still, focus too much upon my breakdown, and looking forward to a point when I would be "better", when the storm would have passed, and, with it, too much of life.

[2] ('Ithaka' from C.P. Cavafy, Collected Poems from C.P. Cavafy. Published by Princeton University Press, 1992. Copyright © C.P. Cavafy. Reproduced by permission of the author c/o Rogers, Coleridge & White Limited, 20 Powis Mews, London W11 1JN.)

Even before I was ill I was aware that my quality of life, or perhaps my balance of life, was not ideal but believed that if I just kept my head down and carried on, somehow I would emerge to a glorious point of fulfilment. I now try to keep in mind the need to accept the rain and learn to be with it and even enjoy it, accepting perhaps that it will never pass and, if I am not careful, I will have reached my Ithaka, blind to the many joys and sumptuous experiences I sailed past on the way, my eyes always fixed upon the mythical horizon, beyond which lay some state in which everything felt whole again.

I was not familiar with the five ways to wellbeing[3] at that time: to learn, connect, give, take notice, and exercise; but without knowing it, I was abiding by their guidance and benefitting from it. Through the course I was learning, connecting, taking notice, and giving – the latter through the interactions with fellow students. During the rest of the week I was endeavouring to be physically active, giving me my exercise. These are the means to maintain wellbeing but at the same time they also operate to enhance it, even to create it if one was, as I felt I was, starting from next-to-zero in this regard.

---

[3] The five ways to wellbeing come from research undertaken by the New Economics Foundation and are much used as a basis for wellbeing projects and a simple guide to self care.

CHAPTER 27

MEANWHILE...

The course provided a source of distraction and direction at a time when family life was changing fast ...

By late 2012 Lucy and I had come to various decisions. We needed to sell the house. We had a massive mortgage which we could not afford with me not earning as I used to. Even when I did return to work it would be a huge burden which would require a commensurately large income. That would then dictate the level and nature of work I would need to be doing. That felt an unnecessary and unhelpful weight to bear. The need to move brought into focus the question of who would move where, and with whom. It is funny that things seem to have come in that order but that's the way I remember it – as if we were unable to make a decision about our relationship in isolation but only in the context of something else. (We had, of course, been trying to work things out for many years by this point, with a lot of couple counselling along the way. It is just that this is how things finally came to a head.)

We concluded that living together was not working – as I have said before, this book is not about the reasons why. What we decided was that we would find a cheaper neighbourhood not too far away, where we could buy two similar houses within walking distance of each other, so that the kids could go easily between the two. We were determined to stay on good terms with each other, for the sake of ourselves as well as the kids; and getting out from under the same roof sooner rather than later seemed to make that a more likely aspiration. We even found two likely looking houses – we would still need a mortgage, but at a much-reduced level.

Telling the kids was surprisingly easy, as it turned out. At Lucy's suggestion, I sat down with them alone to tell them what we had decided, giving her the opportunity to do the same a day or two later – the idea being they could speak freely to either one of us without risking upsetting the other, I think. Their reaction was encouraging. First of all, they recognised that the current situation was making the two of us unhappy, which also impacted them. Secondly, the idea of two houses near each other seemed to preserve the sense of a family unit. Finally, they each had friends whose parents had split up but shared responsibility and got on well with each other, and so they had models they had seen operating in which they could place some trust. 'If it stops you arguing then it's a good thing' was the most memorable response.

In the end, life got in the way of things. It was not until April 2013 that we eventually sold the house by which time financial circumstances had changed, so we ended up buying a house for Lucy and the kids, with me renting round the corner.

When you are trying to recover from anxiety and depression, stability and community are pretty valuable currencies. If I had to plot the things that would be least helpful to a recovery process, separating from your spouse, living apart from your children, moving out of the house you have known for many years, the inevitable social seclusion that results from marital breakdown, finding and furnishing a new home on your own, would all feature close to the top of the list.

It was shit timing – but shit happens. Mental breakdowns and marital breakdowns are, perhaps inevitably, commonly close companions. The way it felt at the time was that it was another layer of onion being stripped away, another part of who I had been, lost. I was losing all I thought I had. And it felt inevitable, like there was nothing I could do to change things. That is almost certainly not true, but it felt that way at the time. I did not feel able to make choices, to make decisions, and so they were being made for me.

This sense of not knowing is captured in some lines I wrote while in France. The quotes included refer back to poems Lucy and I exchanged when we were courting (I do love that word) in the mid-nineties.

Lingering

Years ago, whilst we lingered on your "almost stage",
You told me you needed a lot of looking after.
Brave and young, knowing nothing of life or co-dependency,
I took it as a call to arms, you needed me and so I needed you.

I told you of where I'd been and who I'd seen,
The details you "used to live without".
And apparently managed to portray a family life
of fun and friends and feeling fine,
Skipping over the abuse, the shame and guilt and
feeling fucked.

Sixteen years on like scouts and guides
we have an array of badges down our arms.
Green for the three children, green again for the
three houses, Author, partner, making fire, cooking and
community service. And now to cap it all a mental
and maybe marital breakdown.

I could not care for you enough,
your emotional support I could not provide.
My first and greatest promise I failed

though I tried and tried and tried.
And in that trying I lost myself and all sense
of what I was and wanted to be.
And now am on my own, trying to
rediscover what is me.

We sometimes speak or text or Skype.
You do not know or care with whom I spoke or
what I did, which for me is all I am and do. You want
to know how I feel which I just don't know. Whether I ever
did or mistakenly gave it up for you I yet can't tell.

And I am not sure I want to tell. A part of me craves
your interest and approval, A pat on the back for all my
hard work. But I know it will not come. And I also know
that if I break my back, I must do it for me, or for the earth
Whose back I break too, and not for a badge.

I watch the fire I lit as the embers glow but seem
to ebb away. I could still add more fuel and keep
them burning but it is late and I am tired.
What to do? Fuel it up or let it die?
What are we lingering on the edge of now?

It is no surprise that through this period I found the anxiety, in particular, returning. Some time towards the end of 2012, I gave up trying to cope with it on my own and went back on to medication. I had worked hard to come off it earlier in the year in France but that had been in a very different environment, and there was no sense of shame in accepting that, back in England, with everything that was going on, I needed help once more.

CHAPTER 28

WHAT TO DO ABOUT WORK?

My work had been consistently supportive of me throughout my time away. In the early days, their support in accessing medical help, making appointments, navigating the requirements of health insurers and telling us it was all okay was invaluable to Lucy and me. As time moved on, the gentle and kind visits from my senior partner were a very welcome contact with the outside world and an ongoing connection with my team. And they kept my position open for me for as long as I wanted.

I had had to make a few visits to the office over the near two years I had been absent and each time I was filled with dread and panic. On each occasion, I made arrangements to get collected as quickly as possible from the ground floor and whisked away to a corner room somewhere so as to minimise the risk of seeing anyone. I trembled with anxiety from well before I left the house to start the journey, and this got worse the closer I got to the office vicinity. I would spend much of the short time there in tears and then need to get as far away as possible as quickly as I could before huddling down in a quiet corner of a street somewhere to breathe and try to calm down.

Everyone I did meet was lovely and supportive, and keen to help in any way. I knew I was liked there and had no reason to fear anyone, but fear them I did. It wasn't the individuals but the world of work they represented that scared me. In truth, aside from the very few visits I had to make, and the odd meeting with my senior partner, after a few months away I thought very little about work and the office, largely because whenever I did, it sent me into a downward spiral of anxiety. Whenever the subject of a return to work came up in conversation, my only thought was: I just cannot contemplate going back there yet.

By the beginning of 2013 it was becoming clear that this was a problem that was not going away. It was important that I started to formulate a way to start earning money again, for all the obvious reasons. So that meant a return to work. But I had a complete mental block when I thought about returning to my old firm. It was a vicious circle and the only way I felt able to break it was to take my firm out of the equation – returning to the world of work had to involve something different. I could not work in another capacity, while still a partner in my old firm. So I decided to leave, which I did with effect from April 2013. They were supportive of that and were also kind enough to pay for some sessions with a career coach, Sarah, to help me think about what I would do next.

With Sarah's encouragement and support, I formulated an idea of a consultancy offering advice and support to employers about their people. The idea was that this would utilise my experience as an employment lawyer, as well as my management experience, but with the added insight and perspective gained from my illness, and subsequent study around mental health and the way people think and interact. I felt it was innovative, but also something that I could control in terms of the demands it made of me – I would be able to take on as much or as little as I felt able to do. I was scared, no doubt about it. Scared of meeting people, scared of being relied upon, scared of failure, scared that my fragile state of mind would deteriorate again. Scared of being on my own. Scared of being scared.

One day that summer an image had come to mind that demanded to be written down. I played with it in my head for an hour or so as I travelled across London until, walking down Whitehall, I sat on a wall, took out my notebook and pen and wrote down my thoughts. I saw myself as a burnt-out shell, that my anxiety, which perhaps had been always burning slowly inside me, had burst into a violent inferno in my breakdown, destroying everything within. A terrifying orgy of consumption and destruction burning through my head, my hands, my eyes, my heart, my very life. Now there was just this empty blackened shell of a building which either needed to be knocked down or somehow renovated and restored. I took some solace from my surroundings – the knowledge that large parts of London had once burnt and had been rebuilt with more order and beauty – and from nature, that after natural fires have apparently destroyed all life, slowly new shoots emerge and nature restores herself. I was not without hope.

It was a confusing image, but its lack of refinement perhaps captures the strength of conflicting emotions. As with any stage of life, or any state of health or wellbeing, there was, and is, never a time when certainty or hope reigns supreme. In the darkest days, despair and anxiety did often manage that trick, but recovery is slow and not linear. The graph fluctuates up and down, but the hope is that, plotted over a long enough period, one can discern at least a gentle incline.

So it was, that with Sarah urging me on and assuring me I could do it, I slowly and cautiously set about making contact with some of the more friendly of my old contacts and clients. Several people, it turned out, were pleased to hear from me again, happy to buy me coffee, and interested to hear what I was planning to do. One or two of them even asked me to help them with some issues, and paid me small sums for doing so. But it was very early on in that process that one old friend and contact asked me whether I had spoken to Matt Dean. I hadn't and, very quickly, contact was arranged.

Matt, it turned out, had been an employment lawyer but had got tired of dealing with the rubbish that comes out of dysfunctional workplaces, the bullying, harassment, discrimination claims, and much else besides. While dealing with such claims provided a good income for lawyers, he saw more value, more purpose, in helping organisations create the sort of culture where those problems did not arise, or at least where their number was reduced – creating kinder, fairer, and more productive workplaces. Over the course of a couple of phone calls we established enough common purpose to know we wanted to work together and in October I formally joined the team.

At the time I was still very unsure of myself, unsure how many hours a week I would feel able to work as well as anxious about having the weight of expectations and targets upon me. Matt and Victoria (Matt's wife and the Byrne of their company byrne·dean) were very understanding of that, and happy to agree to accommodate my needs and uncertainties.

I also knew that I wanted to continue with a focus in mental health-related issues. At the time this took the form of enrolling for a three-year Masters course in psychotherapy and counselling which began that October – the natural follow-on course from the foundation course I had completed earlier in the year. I had been accepted on the course before even hearing of byrne·dean. Again it was part-time, with classes on Fridays.

I think it was probably only the second Friday of the course when I found myself caught between being late for a lecture and a client on the phone wanting advice. I realised there and then that trying to combine the two would severely test my anxiety and time-management skills. So early on in the course, it was easy to back out. The purpose of the course was to train you to be a counsellor. I had enrolled because I was not sure where my future career lay. In that instant I realised that, for now at least, I did not want to be a counsellor, I had found a place to work that felt right, and, therefore, the obvious thing was to abandon the course, which I duly did.

At the same time, I realised that I could maintain and develop an interest in mental health in a different way, working with employers to increase awareness of mental health and wellbeing. Partly this is born of a desire to help people avoid what happened to me, but partly it is about the straightforward fact that people who are well perform better, communicate better, create less conflict, are more creative, and have more enjoyable lives at the same time. I have also now trained to be a coach, on the basis that the opportunity for people to talk openly about whatever issues they are dealing with is a way to maintain positive mental health – perhaps this reflects the instinct that took me into a counselling course but from a different angle.

By the end of that year, 2013, I was working pretty much every day and largely coping with it. Our Christmas party (the first work Christmas do I had attended since 2010) was in a dining room above a pub in Victoria, gathering together those who worked all the time in the business, as well as people who did a bit here and there, and others who were simply good friends of the business. As I joined in the celebrations, still meeting some people for the first time, I had a huge sense of belonging, of having found a group of kindred spirits committed to doing valuable, purposeful work, and of feeling safe with them.

CHAPTER 29

MY TREATMENT

I have talked about aspects of my treatment as I have gone along, but I am conscious that the detail may have got lost at times in the wider narrative. What follows is what I did, and is not offered as any kind of guide to what anyone else should do. Everyone has their own experience and must listen to themselves and their doctor(s), and follow their advice.

One thing I would plead for is that, if you ever need it, you do seek help. Once you recognise that something is not right you have taken a hugely important first step. You owe it to yourself to do something about it – you are worth it. If you carry on doing the same stuff that has got you to that place, then there is only one way that things are going to head. And mental health problems are an illness. If you had cancer, or diabetes, or failing vision, you would not try to deal with it on your own. You wouldn't think you can sort it out without expert help. Mental health is no different. Life is hard. It is no surprise, and no shame, that sometimes we find it hard to cope. The only shame is in not seeking the help you need.

Once back in England in 2011 my first port of call was my doctor. He was (and is) everything I could have hoped for in a general practitioner. I can still remember sitting in his surgery room terrified of what was happening to me, while he looked at me with kind and understanding eyes, clearly aware that I was far from well, but giving me the reassurance that I was safe, he would look after me; it was okay.

It is well worth keeping in touch with your doctor. There are the practical reasons – sick notes and prescriptions – and there is another source of support, someone else to talk to. And, on a purely practical front, as I have said earlier, insurers, or others, might expect you to have regular appointments with your doctor and question how ill you really are if you don't.

My psychiatrist saw me at least fortnightly at the outset, was fairly ever-present in the Priory, and then saw me every month or so when I was in England, gradually reducing in regularity until the back end of 2013. He was "in charge". It was he who made the initial diagnosis, he who admitted me to the Priory, he who prescribed medication and therapy, he who guided me as to appropriate levels of activity over the months. He gave me the confidence that he had seen people like me before, lots of them, and although the road ahead was not always going to be easy or predictable, he told me that we would walk it together as far as I needed him with me, and even when I ventured forth on my own, he would always be available.

In my view there are three aspects to treatment for anxiety and depression – dealing with the symptoms, dealing with the cause, and trying to prevent a relapse or recurrence.

Everyone's symptoms are different and everyone will have different levels of tolerance. There are myriad different possible treatments for the symptoms of anxiety and depression. In my case I would not have been able to carry on living without prescribed anti-anxiety / depression medication. There are lots of tips and techniques I picked up along the way – meditation, breathing exercises, mindfulness, rest, massage, reiki, and more besides – but none got close to dealing with the agony of my anxiety for anything other than short periods. I know there is stigma and distrust around psychiatric medication – and this is probably not helped by the limited understanding of why particular drugs seem to help. But to my mind if you have any other kind of illness and a doctor recommends medicine, most people would take it (some wouldn't, for a whole range of different reasons, and I respect that). There is no difference with drugs that are prescribed to deal with the symptoms of anxiety and depression.

I am someone who tends not to reach for the medicine cabinet whenever I have a headache or other pain. This is not from some sense of distrust of medication or desire to suffer, but rather that the pain is telling me something which I probably ought to hear.

With my anxiety, the pain was just too great to even think about trying to cope without something. I knew there might be side-effects but all drugs have possible side-effects. My doctor suggested we would try something at a certain dose – low to begin with – to see if I had any problematic side-effects and whether it was helping. If it did not seem to help, or if the side-effects were a problem, then we could try something else.

My initial prescription was 10mg a day of citalopram. Citalopram is one of the SSRI (Selective Serotonin Reuptake Inhibitors) class of drugs, designed to reduce the body's reabsorption of serotonin, thereby increasing the amount available. Like all drugs it has a long list of potential side-effects, and there are a number of drugs you must not take in combination with it. 10mg is a low dose but you start low and build up gradually, monitoring both side-effects and effectiveness until you reach a point where the balance between effectiveness and side-effects feels right – which is based on a discussion between you and the doctor.

Because it is designed to dull the extremes of depression and anxiety, a side-effect is that it will reduce, or numb, your overall emotional responsiveness. Too high a dose and it will deprive you of any real emotion. So you want to get to a point where it makes the anxiety and depression bearable but you still retain some sense of what's going on for you. You also need to bear in mind that the drugs will often take at least a fortnight to start having a noticeable effect on your mood.

My doctor gradually increased the dose by instalments of 10mg until I was at 40mg a day. When I came off the drugs, I did so again very gradually, reducing the dose by no more than 10mg a month at a time, and then, when I was down to 10mg a day, taking that alternate days for a period until I reduced to nothing at all. It is vital that you follow medical advice when taking drugs of this kind, that you monitor yourself for side-effects and discuss them with the doctor, and that you only come off the drugs under supervision from the doctor.

I came off the drugs in the summer of 2012, but went back on them later in the year. By the summer of 2015 though, I felt that I was ready to try to come off the drugs again. I was fairly stable and wanted to see if I could cope without them. I had been on them again for more than two years and was conscious that they were suppressing my emotions generally. I wanted to see whether the benefit of having a richer all-round emotional experience was worth the additional anxiety that I might experience without the drugs. A year and a half later, a combination of different factors was creating anxiety problems again and I went back on to medication.

As I have said, medication is just part of the equation – it arrests the decline. It stabilises you. It does not make you better. In my experience, getting better is something that takes time, talking therapy and, potentially, adjustments to the way you both live and think about your life.

There are many different kinds of talking therapy. At its heart, and whatever the theory and methodology, psychotherapy is about exploring the thoughts of the patient or client – what thoughts, memories, beliefs are going on that are affecting the way the client sees the world in a way that is unhelpful to them. Some approaches focus on conscious thoughts, some on unconscious thought patterns, others look to untap long suppressed, and otherwise inaccessible, thoughts and memories.

At one end of the spectrum CBT will seek to identify unhelpful thinking patterns and challenge the client to create more helpful thinking patterns. It is not necessarily concerned with why the client thinks like that, other than perhaps as a means to understand the pattern itself.

At the other end of the spectrum, psychoanalysis of the kind practised by Freud and still common today, will require the client to explore her / his earliest and deepest memories, emotions, and experiences in order to try to understand the individual's subconscious. Often in psychoanalysis the focus will be on identifying where the individual's psychic development has been arrested and / or disrupting the defence mechanisms the individual has subconsciously put in place to protect against psychic wounds. The theory is that those mechanisms are proving themselves to be ineffective in allowing the individual to have his or her needs met.

Different forms of practice will have different demands in terms of length of treatment and regularity of session. CBT, for example, will tend to be weekly, perhaps for 6–20 sessions. It is project focused – the therapist and client will agree what they are looking to deal with and create a plan to do that. Some of the work will be done in sessions, but most of it will be down to the client to do between sessions. There are also online CBT resources and numerous self-help books. Psychoanalysis, on the other hand, can last for years and years (often a whole lifetime), and may involve several sessions in a week.

Although there are purists out there who will strictly adhere to one approach to therapy, eschewing all others, many therapists adopt a blended approach. While their practice may be based in one or another tradition, they will draw from others in a more integrative approach. Many will use elements of what is called a person-centred approach, where the therapist is non-directive and allows the client to dictate the subject matter of discussion in the sessions, encouraging the client to reflect on what (s)he is saying, drawing connections, asking questions.

I had never really paused to reflect on the extent of my subconscious thoughts and how much they influenced my behaviours and reactions to events and people. I had, I guess, just taken all that as being who I was, without wondering why that was the case, or recognising any negative impacts, or contemplating the possibility of change. For me, therefore, the weeks spent in the Priory were revelatory. I found the group CBT sessions very helpful in giving me a starting point for ongoing work. I am not sure that the therapy which followed on from the Priory would have been as effective without that initial grounding.

Over the years, I have had three therapists. The first was very much CBT-based and was recommended by my psychiatrist. I sort of drifted out of that in the end, feeling that I was not really connecting with her, or perhaps she with me.

The stays in France meant that there were periods where I was not "in" therapy, but in late 2012, I think, I decided to re-engage. I wanted someone who would be less directive than the CBT approach I had experienced to date. Again, I turned to my psychiatrist for advice, and he put me in touch with a chap who I then saw on and off for more than a year. His approach is integrative or eclectic, using whatever techniques appear to be most helpful for the client, and is very much person-centred.

He was happy to work via Skype if I was away in France, which many therapists would not do. He helped me undoubtedly, unpicking and exploring the issues and my thoughts about them. By the end I was feeling that I was able to do a lot of the work myself – that as I was speaking, I was analysing my own words and thoughts and resolving them. I also felt that our relationship was becoming too matey. It was a commitment of time and money that I was beginning to feel was not justified.

After several months not attending therapy, my search for my third therapist was primarily based on her approach. I felt that previously, I had been looking for answers, looking for understanding that would make me feel better, that there was a truth that was obtainable that would make sense and would enable me to live calmly, without my anxiety. I began to realise that this approach, this search, was not proving successful and was not making the anxiety go away. Rather, perhaps, I ought to be more accepting of my anxiety, more open to uncertainty, more interested in questions than in answers.

I therefore sought someone who used existential approaches in their work. Existentialism is a philosophy that emphasises individual existence, freedom, and choice. It is the view that humans define their own meaning in life, and try to make rational decisions, despite existing in an irrational universe. There is a strong emphasis on how the individual relates to their world, it emphasises the choices we have about what we do, how we react, how we feel, and does not seek to cure people, but to help them find a satisfactory way of living that works for them.

Recommendation from a doctor or a friend is often a good way of finding a therapist. But you can also do your research yourself. Although there are no formal qualifications or certifications required to set yourself up as a therapist or counsellor, most reputable practitioners in the UK will be members of either the UK Council for Psychotherapy or the British Association for Psychotherapy and Counselling.

Both organisations have training requirements for their members and so membership does provide assurance of training as well as adherence to the professional standards of the organisation. Both have websites that allow you to search by area of practice, by the nature of the problem you are facing, and by geographic location. You can then go through the therapists your search reveals and see what you think. Sometimes what (s)he says about their work and style will be enough to remove them from your shortlist. If you end up with a few to choose between, most will be happy to have an introductory phone call for free to see how you get on. This will be a two-way decision – the therapist may conclude that (s)he does not think (s)he will be able to work with you, but that is rare, and there would usually need to be good reason for rejecting someone at that stage. Internet research like this was how I found my third therapist with whom I worked for over two years.

It is worth stating that the choice of therapist should not be based on whether you like the person – what you need to find is someone who can help you – that may well make you feel very uncomfortable at times. If you are just looking for someone to have a nice chat with, who will tell you nice things and make you feel good about yourself, you are better off getting a friend than a therapist – it will be much cheaper, too!

Therapy tends to take place at the therapist's place of work. Some will work from their house, some from rooms they have hired in shared office space, some will work in collaboration with other therapists and have a therapy centre. Location is something you need to think about when making your choice. Therapy is a commitment and you want to avoid, therefore, somewhere that is going to be inconvenient or hard to get to on those days when you really feel you can't be bothered – keep the hurdles-to-attendance to a minimum where you can.

Wherever it takes place, the room is likely to be pretty neutral. The therapist will generally want to create a space that is calm and not distracting, and which says very little about them. The sessions are about the client.

Therapy sessions last for "the therapist's hour", which generally means 50 minutes. The timing is strict. The session starts and ends at the appointed time, determined by the therapist's clock. You will agree a day of the week and a time and usually that will be the same every week – so again try not to agree to something that is likely to prove tricky. The same time slot in the same place every time are part of the therapeutic frame the therapist will try to create around the sessions.

As a result, some will be quite reluctant to agree to swap session times around, other than in real emergencies.

During the first session the therapist will explain their method of working and will start to establish that therapeutic frame. This will include times and venues, but also fee arrangements and holiday periods. It is common for therapists to require you to pay for sessions even when you are not able to attend. They will let you know when they will be on holiday (when you won't have to pay) but the deal is that every other week they are there, available for you at the allotted time, whether you choose to take advantage of that or not. This certainly encourages you to attend and to avoid cancelling sessions at short notice.

Most therapists operate privately and will charge you for their services. Some employers may offer counselling as part of the employee benefit package, often through private medical cover or employee assistance programmes. Provision under such schemes tends to be limited to a small number of sessions. Some employers are now employing their own in-house counsellors, available to staff on demand. That remains rare. It is, however, always worth asking your employer what, if any, provision they fund.

There are sometimes local charities which provide free or subsidised counselling. It is worth asking around to find out about what exists in your area.

Some therapy relationships last for years and years, others are more short-term. What you are looking for in a therapist may change, as well. At the outset, when I was still very vulnerable and unsure of myself, I wanted someone who would be quite directive, give me stuff to work on, set an agenda to some extent, and tell me what she thought. My CBT therapist was right for me then. Later, I wanted to be more reflective, with less direction (and less homework), a relationship that somehow felt more equal. That required a different personality and a different style of approach.

What happens in a therapy session will depend very much upon you, the style of practice of the therapist, and how you interact. You will often have the choice of sitting in a chair or lying on a couch. Each has benefits and drawbacks. Being in a chair means you see the therapist and tend to have more sense of him or her as a person and are aware of their attention on you and their reactions to things you say (albeit these will usually be quite limited). It is a more familiar way to have a conversation, which is both good and bad. It may be less intimidating but can encourage you to adopt a more conversational approach to the session.

On the couch, you are unlikely to have eye contact with the therapist, may not be able to see him or her at all, and you are very clearly in a therapeutic pose. It can be easier to immerse yourself in your own thoughts and feelings, but it can also leave you feeling quite alone. Every now and then there is the worry that the therapist is not paying you any attention and has, in fact, drifted off to sleep! In a funny way, despite the lack of eye contact, the couch can make one feel much more protected and held by the therapist. It is a more vulnerable position to be in and the fact that you can adopt that pose creates that sense of being looked after. That is my experience at any rate.

What you talk about will again be determined by the nature of the therapy. In CBT, the discussion will be structured by the therapist to a large extent. With more person-centred approaches the client will be left to talk about anything they want, or not to talk at all. If the therapist feels that the topic is not helpful then (s)he may ask questions about why the client wants to talk about it but that is not common, more likely it is that the therapist will assume there is a reason and will allow that reason to emerge.

Sometimes I will approach a therapy session with a clear sense of wanting to talk about an issue that is troubling me. Sometimes it will begin more with a reflection of events and feelings since the previous session. Sometimes I have no real idea of what I am going to talk about but just start talking about whatever thoughts occur to me. Quite often I worry that I am not doing it right, and then remind myself there is no right way, just my way.

I find that most sessions will leave me challenged to a greater or lesser extent. I will often be emotional during a session, crying, not out of sadness, but because of exploring the core of me, of being really challenged. Sometimes this can leave me quite unsettled and vulnerable for the rest of the day as thoughts and feelings settle into a slightly new order. I find it is best not to head straight from therapy to a client meeting! At the end of the day, like most things, what you get out of it will depend to a large extent on what you put into it, and if I am distracted or feeling flat and lethargic at the start of a session, that will often be reflected in what happens in the session.

The focus in therapy is you: your thoughts, your feelings, your experiences. It does not matter, and you generally won't know, whether your therapist has had similar experiences. I can look at someone middle aged and assume that (s)he has similar life experience but (s)he may not be married, may not have had kids, might still be living with her / his parents – I have no idea. You have to trust the therapist to be able to hold you and your issues. If you are concerned they can't, then talk about it, and maybe think about a change.

Pills and therapy were a very important part of my recovery. But there is a whole lot more to my treatment – engaging with the world in different ways, through working in a shop, volunteering at school, seeing friends, attending courses, and starting to work. They were all hugely important in rebuilding my confidence, sense of purpose, and identity. Taking care of myself was important, as was exercise. My various DIY projects also formed a big part of the process. So did gardening. As well as the exercise, there is something about being grounded, present, purposeful, nurturing, and absorbed that gardening can provide.

There is an increasing amount of interest in the effectiveness of gardening as a therapeutic exercise in itself. My brother Andy runs a project called Grozone (www.grozone.org.uk) – a community project created around an open space. The majority of people who attend are volunteers in one form or another, who come there because they get something from it. There is a community there for those that lack contact with people – often something that can be the cause of, or caused by, mental health problems. And there is activity.

The team grow vegetables and fruit. Much of this is in beds that are specially designed to be accessible to those in wheelchairs. They build things – everything on the site was built by team members, ranging from a compost toilet with wheelchair access to a covered kitchen area. They cook – on a regular basis there will be a meal prepared by team members which is then shared with whoever is there that day. Much of the food eaten is grown on site. Stuff happens and there is a purpose to the activity but more important than the end product is the community, the coming together of people to create the end product. It is about the journey again, rather than Ithaka herself.

In terms of the ways to wellbeing, the volunteers get ample doses of learning, connection, exercise, giving, and taking notice. Increasingly, local doctors are suggesting to patients that they spend time at Grozone rather than take home a prescription for medication – because it is seen to work. It may not be right for the most severe cases, but, for mild to moderate anxiety and depression, it is proving a hugely effective tool.

I said at the outset of this chapter that there were three aspects to treatment: the symptoms, towards which medication is directed; the underlying causes of the problem(s) you are experiencing; and then preventing relapse / recurrence. Therapy is aimed at the latter two, and my distinction between the two of them is a little false. It is rarely (if ever) the case that someone experiences significant anxiety or depression (for example), has treatment, and then recovers back to where they were before. An experience of this kind changes you, as do all experiences all the time. One of my therapists encouraged me to think of my breakdown as a breakthrough to a new level of understanding and experience. There was not, could not, and should not have been any sense of getting back to where I was because that was not a safe place as it turned out. To "get back" would be to ignore so much of what I have learnt about myself.

My life changed in almost every aspect. I decided not to try to return to my old job, a decision I believe was right at the time, but need not be forever. I separated from Lucy, moved house, and also, in the process, lost my relationship with organised religion. I cannot expect to get back to where I was, and any recovery plan that set that as a goal would be doomed to failure. Other people will have less background change going on, and so returning to a state in which they can cope with what they coped with before, might be a realistic goal.

The fundamental lesson I have learnt is to be aware of my feelings and to respect them – I could say that I ignored them before, but that implies I was even aware of them, which I am not sure is true. A realistic estimation for what recovery looks like for me, therefore, is being able to exist with my feelings – that, for enough of the time to be bearable, I can interact with the world and the people in it; contribute to it in a meaningful way; be respectful of myself and other people; and be as much of the father, friend, colleague and partner that other people need and I can manage. In that, recovery and the prevention of relapse are very much one and the same. The awareness and care that is required for continued recovery is the same as that required to avert relapse.

CHAPTER 30

THE VIEW FIVE YEARS ON

It would be lovely were I able to end with how I lived happily ever after, anxiety and depression behind me. But it is not like that.

It has been more than five years since my breakdown. For cancer survivors that is a milestone, and the same is true for me in a sense. I started my diary when I was first ill so I could remember what happened day-to-day, and because it helped me to write stuff down, to articulate what I was feeling. I had a vague idea it might have other uses at some stage.

The diary had sat in my documents folder for the best part of five years, mostly unread, but reminding me every now and then of the need to go back to it and try to make some sense of it – for me and, perhaps, for others. In late 2015, I was in my weekly counselling session and, out of nowhere, while talking and thinking about a feeling of having moved into a more positive frame of mind, a thought came to me that felt like a title for a book – one day I walked out without my anxiety. So it felt like the time had come to revisit the diary.

That title did not stand the test of time or realism. Although there are days when I don't really notice my anxiety, it would have given the false impression that one day I did just leave it all behind. I didn't. Life is inherently anxious to a greater or lesser degree and I try to be honest and self-aware enough to accept that – and kind enough to myself too. Indeed, being open to anxiety is to embrace life to an extent. But at the same time, I do experience it more fiercely than I would like. I hope that my process of recovery is not yet at an end, that the fluctuating curve of recovery still shows an overall upward trend.

I am regularly reminded of how far I have come. I mentioned the firework display in 2011 and how it terrified me and left me in a desperate state. Where I now live there is another school at the end of the road that has an even more impressive display every year. You can pay to go in, or you can stand on the pavement next to the school and watch for free. I have suffered every November and New Year (now that we have expanded our national pyrotechnic horizons) since that first one in 2011. Last November, however, I decided to test myself and joined the crowds on the pavement at the end of my road. I was on my own. I wanted it that way so that I could run away if need be, and because I spend a lot of my time on my own. Anyway, I actually enjoyed the display. My heart did not race, I did not shake in terror and I stayed for the whole thing and had a proud smile on my face as I walked home.

I often find myself at Vauxhall station in London where there is an interchange between the overground trains and the Victoria Tube line. Often, as I walk down the steps I remember how, not that long ago, this would have been the point at which I broke my journey for a few minutes to breathe, relax, congratulate myself on getting this far, and then summon up the mental strength to face the next stage. Yet now, I march confidently off to the Tube station without a second thought. And a good job too because I no longer leave myself an extra half-hour or more for every journey in case of emergencies.

I have done a couple of trips to New York to deliver some training on mental health awareness in the workplace. On the first occasion, the trip had been set up a few months in advance and there was a voice in my head somewhere scoffing at the very idea that I was going to just pack a suitcase, get on a plane, on my own, to America, stay in a hotel on my own for a week and talk to several bunches of people I had never met before. I think that voice assumed that, somehow, it wouldn't really happen, and perhaps that stopped me worrying about it. But the trip wasn't cancelled, so I packed my case and I enjoyed pretty much every minute of it, and allowed myself a pat on the back at the end.

Social occasions are less fraught too. I have mentioned before how wonderfully musical the kids are (and Lucy too). Gina and Jude's piano teacher organises regular soirées in someone's house where various of the kids she teaches come, with their parents, to play pieces, some much planned, some more impromptu. Not so long ago, Lucy had suggested that we all go to one of these evenings together. It was at the end of a working week, I was probably quite tired and was feeling very anxious about going to a place I did not know, with people whose names I couldn't remember, who did not make me feel safe. It may be that it reminded me too much of our previous life all together – a couple and a house, comfortable and confident enough in themselves to throw open their doors and welcome a group of other families.

As the time approached, I decided I could not face it so texted Lucy to say so, but she asked whether I could at least go with them to help carry in various instruments – a cello or two and some djembe drums. She said that I could just take the gear in then quietly disappear. Unfortunately, it did not work out that way. By the time I had carried the instruments in, the door had been closed behind me and I was being offered a drink and was enveloped in conversation. I started to panic. I could feel my heart beginning to race, my mind on overdrive, breathlessness, and nausea rising. I could have said that I was not feeling well and made my excuses, but something stopped me.

After a few minutes, we took our seats in the living room, various of us perched on arms of chairs or on the floor. The music washed over me. All I could feel was the rising tension in my body. I managed to stay for our kids' planned pieces and then had to make a dash for the door. I whispered to Lucy that I had to go and left her to make my excuses. The walk home was about a mile. It was still light. I was crying and stumbling, shaking and massively distraught. I kept trying to focus on getting home, repeatedly working out how much further I had to go, but becoming increasingly overwhelmed. Would I be able to make it back in time?

Eventually I gave in, sat down on a wall at the side of the pavement and let the tears and waves of panic engulf me. I felt desperately alone, yet terrified of anyone coming to my aid. If I saw someone walking towards me I would try to gather myself together for the few seconds it would take them to pass me before I could release it all again. All I wanted was someone who I knew and could feel safe with to come and put their arms around me, take me home and tell me it was okay. Eventually I made it home.

More recently, I have been to a couple more of those evenings and felt fine, have enjoyed the evening, and surprised myself at my ability to chatter with the other kids and parents, joke, engage in discussions and keep it together. It is, undoubtedly, progress.

My flat is variously a safe haven and a place of depressing isolation. It is in a grand, late-Victorian, house that has been converted into flats. Mine is in the basement. When Lucy and I separated in 2013 and I started renting, I looked at what might be available to buy in the area within a reasonable budget, once my finances had stabilised a little. I saw this flat and thought that it would work and was just about affordable. I did not think much more about it until a year or so later. I was starting to think I might be in a position to buy somewhere and, again, saw a for sale board outside the property.

It was just right. It turned out that there had been a buyer lined up but he had dithered and dallied and eventually pulled out, so it was back on the market, at the same price as a year before. Much like the French house, it felt destined. As if it had been waiting for me, and I agreed to buy. It was in a state of renovation – about half complete. I would be able to finish the job off and make myself a home.

There was some building work required to create an additional bedroom, re-arrange bathrooms, and knock through here and there to adjust the space to what worked for me, living here on my own for much of the time, but having the three kids to stay on a regular basis. The structural and plumbing work needed professionals. The rest I took on myself. Foolishly, I had largely completed the wholesale redecoration after the main building work before I decided to have the electrics tested, only to be told the existing system needed to be completely renewed. All the work I had done to clear the debris and dust from the building work, and decorate throughout, was undone as the electrician set about replacing every wire and fitting in the flat.

My anxiety was pushed to its limits as, for several weeks, I lived and tried to work in the flat, around the ongoing work. As the days passed, the electrician went from room to room, reducing inexorably the space I had left to occupy behind the advancing line of debris and destruction. He would fill the flat with a cacophony of his own singing, the radio he insisted on playing, and the deafening sound of power tools ripping through my walls. My haven was reduced, bit by bit, until I had one corner of my living room to occupy. When that too was taken away I took to working in coffee shops, but that was limited because of the need to refer to papers and books that were in the flat and too voluminous to cart around with me everywhere. When he had finished the technical work, I couldn't wait to get him out and reclaim the place to myself. I was happy to do the remaining work – if only to have some peace and control back.

I never felt able to tell him just what effect he was having on me. I think that I assumed he must at least have been capable of recognising that for himself. I feared the sense of confrontation that I believed would necessarily arise if I tried to ask him to adjust how he was working to accommodate my needs. And therein lies one of the old problems.

In one of the psychodrama sessions in the Priory, we had begun with everyone standing up and being asked to put our right hands on the right shoulder of someone we felt most connected to, and then our left hand on the left shoulder of someone else, and then touch feet with yet another person. I ended up precariously balanced on one leg, stretching with the other leg and my arms to reach the three people, while accommodating those reaching out to touch me. The therapist observed my position and asked whether I was comfortable – clearly not – and whether I often felt like this – very much so. She pointed to everyone else in the group who seemed to have found quite comfortable poses and suggested that I might ask people to shuffle around a little to ease my discomfort. Of course it worked, without inconveniencing anyone.

Learning to recognise my own wants and needs, and to express them, remains one of my biggest challenges. Too often, still, I find myself having agreed to things I don't want to do because it is what someone else wants. The point at which I do challenge it and say what I want, feels very much like vomiting, that the expression of what I want is having to be violently retched out of me. In the same way that vomiting can leave you feeling cleansed and stable, I am left in the same state – the process may be deeply unpleasant, but the outcome feels right. I still have to learn a kinder, less dramatic way of making and expressing my own choices. The words of my coach, 'But Richard, what do you want?,' still echo.

Another echo is a mantra from the Priory – "Mind the gap". We all have a tendency to picture how we would like our lives to be and then see how they actually are (focusing inevitably on the negative aspects). As we ruminate on the gap, it widens, and our dissatisfaction and depression increase. It happens when I think about people in relationships. I make huge assumptions about how perfect and happy those relationships must be, and wish that I had the same. I also experience it in the context of people doing things and having fun experiences (Facebook is a great source of dissatisfaction). Then I beat myself up about how I am not doing the same, filling myself with guilt and a degree of self-loathing as a result. I do still feel that I am living, if not half a life, at least not a complete one.

I will try to reassure myself that things are okay, and that I am still very much in recovery from what was (is?) a significant illness. I am trying to do my best, and most of the time I seem to cope. Sometimes it all becomes too much. Not so long ago I was coming home from work on a Thursday with a heavy bag of work stuff over my shoulder. The kids come to stay on Thursdays, so I had stopped off to buy supper and other food shopping. As a result, I had two heavy bags of shopping to go with my work bag. The bus stop at the end of my road was closed so I had longer than normal to walk with my assorted burdens. I finally got home, started to unpack the shopping and put it away, and dropped a four-pint milk carton on the floor ... It tipped me over the edge. I tried to tell myself there was, after all, no point crying over spilt milk! But cry I did. All I wanted was for someone to smile and say don't worry, sit down and let me sort this out. But there was no one there.

That isolation also means it's only ever up to me to look after myself, which I don't always do. There are times when I cannot be bothered to cook a meal and so go without, knowing all the while that is not good for me. I don't always get the sleep I need, and I drink too much. Sometimes I find the whole business of having to make decisions about everything overwhelming. I just want someone else to decide for a change.

But I am learning. A few weeks before the spilt milk, I had a particularly dark day in mid-April. I had had problems with my knee all year which had stopped me exercising since very early

January. It is the same knee that I had an operation on several years ago. Finally, I had an appointment with a specialist who confirmed, subject to the results of an MRI scan, that I had torn my meniscus which would require an operation to repair. On one level, it was helpful to know what was wrong, and that I had not been making up the pain for the last several months. On another, it brought a depressing anticipation of weeks or months more of not being able to exercise, and of pain.

Over the previous months, my plans to improve my stamina and work towards a half marathon had been abandoned, while I jealously watched the growing numbers of runners out everywhere as the weather improved.

At the same time, I was very tired from a long week at work, and frustrated about not having been able to resolve a work issue. I had had counselling in the morning, which often leaves me vulnerable, and I was facing a weekend without the kids, and without any plans to see anyone – a long, lonely weekend of brooding.

I felt very low, despairing at times, and often tearful. I tried to distract myself by working late and by buying some new music, but it only postponed the inevitable. I found solace, as I do too regularly, in a bottle of wine and a discount pizza from the supermarket, because I could not be bothered to make an effort to cook something, and had convinced myself I did not deserve anything more exciting for supper.

I did email my brothers and my dad to tell them about my knee.

The following day, however, was another day. Partly through their efforts and partly through mine, I arranged to see some friends. My dad telephoned (he never phones me) to ask if I needed any help with shopping. I didn't, but it was so kind of him to offer, and so nice to hear another human voice expressing concern for me. And I took myself off for a bike ride for a couple of hours, wearing sports kit to underline to myself that this was exercise.

I knew that I had been neglecting myself and knew that exercise would be a good place to start, but it was touch-and-go whether I actually went. There were many other things I could have pretended were more important to do, and there was no one else here to tell me just to get out on my bike, but I went, and by lunchtime I felt so much better.

I came back and shaved and showered, and put on some different clothes that I had not worn for a while, not for anyone else's benefit but just because I felt like a change, something new. I made something to eat – nothing fancy but a change from a slab of cheese or ham stuffed inside some form of bread with a load of crisps on the side which would be my default option. I felt more confident, more empowered, more happy. It really was a few very simple steps that made the change, and no one was going to make them but me.

I have not been able to silence the nagging voice in my ear that says I must be doing something all the time. That somehow, I have to be able to give an account of my time and show how I have used it wisely. When I do let myself just be, rather than do, it is almost always rewarding and restorative.

I have been "back at work" for several years now. It is not a regular office job, in that I have a lot of autonomy over where and how I spend my time. Aside from general HR advisory support, I do some conflict resolution work, encouraging people to understand and resolve their issues through conversation rather than confrontation or litigation, and then an increasing amount of training and consulting work around mental health and wellbeing. This is about helping employers create environments and cultures in which people understand their own wellbeing, are alive to its importance and to the warning signs of problems developing. We want them to talk about their wellbeing safely, and know that there is support in place to help if they need it.

All of this requires of me a vulnerability and openness that I never used as a lawyer. I talk freely about my health problems.

This was difficult at first, but I am more confident about it now. As part of the Lord Mayor's This is Me in the City campaign to encourage people to talk about their mental health, I was featured in *City AM*, one of London's daily newspapers. I am now on the steering committee of the group. I campaign about the stigma surrounding mental health, and I know that the way to break stigma is to inform people, and enable people to tell their stories. It makes sense therefore for me to tell mine. In doing so, I am careful to stay (just) within the bounds of where I feel safe, but every now and then, something happens to take you out of the safe place ...

I was delivering some training one day at a client's offices and the lady introducing me said that she had not had any personal mental health problems but would share something about her father. She told of his struggles with depression and how, for a long time, he contemplated and actively planned suicide. She finished by saying that although it was a difficult period for all concerned, she now felt they were through the worst and that she had her dad back. And then I was supposed to start my piece, except I couldn't because her words had made me think of my own kids and their perspective of my illness, and my eyes were full of tears. I took a minute to compose myself, which I think went unnoticed, and all was well.

That vulnerability is really just an acknowledgement of what is there within me, was always there within me. But I chose to keep it hidden as part of my professional and (all too often) personal bravado. The same is true of my anxiety, I think. Anxiety is part of life. Letting it show is part of being vulnerable. I have learnt that being vulnerable is okay and, as a result, I just show my anxiety more than I ever used to – or, put another way, my anxiety shows itself more than I ever used to allow.

I was challenged recently by a close friend who knew me in work long before I was ill – she remarked that I seemed to be defining myself by reference to having been ill. She was talking primarily about my work but the same could be true of most aspects of my life. I am wary of things, I am careful of myself, I say no too often when I should be saying yes – and I use that "should" word too often when a fairer word would be "could". I also struggle with a sense of identity. Being a lawyer gives you a clear sense of identity, as does being a husband and father. Much of how I talk about myself is still by reference to the past – 'I used to be a lawyer, I used to be married to Lucy.' As Neil Diamond once put it, "Used to be's don't count any more, they just lay on the floor 'til we sweep them away."

I am happiest when I can accept myself for what I am – not what I used to be, not what I do, and not what badge I wear, but what I am. That is hard, though, when the primary reference point for so many years was how others perceived me, pleasing them and doing what they wanted. It requires the re-wiring of decades of thinking and instinctive habit. Larkin, in his poem 'Aubade', talks of how "An only life can take so long to climb clear of its wrong beginnings, and may never".

It remains, therefore, an ongoing project, this living business. I have not got it cracked yet by any means. But I think have a better understanding now than I ever did of myself, of how I think and behave, and why. That insight is the key to exercising choice. On many different levels, it is the key to being kind to yourself, which only you can do. And that also requires acceptance, of who you are and how things are, without constantly focusing on that damn gap. When I feel stressed or anxious, I have learnt to recognise it for what it is, to stop and to think about what it is that is making me feel that way and to ask myself whether those feelings are justified. I can look for alternative ways of reacting to the situation, and, sometimes, just accept that that is what I am feeling, and look after myself as best as I can.

As well as caring for myself at times of heightened anxiety, there is the day-to-day nurturing, which really boils down to those ways to wellbeing, or variations thereon. Connection and talking to people makes you feel good – and letting them be kind to you when they want to, rather than pushing that away. Exercise, giving, learning, and taking notice – while walking on the common in the early summer, with Steph (getting exercise and connection), I was enthralled by the different tones of green in the leaves on the trees. I was lost in the wonder of the variety of nature – and moments like that – self-actualising in the language of Maslow – are a great form of medication, and confirmation that you are still alive.

I would have liked to be able to end with some fine words that somehow unravelled life's great mystery. I can't, of course. What I can offer is hope. Everyone who suffers mental turmoil will have their own experience and, hopefully, will find their own way through it. Seldom, I fear, do they emerge suddenly into a golden land of happiness and understanding. But most will emerge, changed and bruised, no doubt, but wiser. Give it time, and be kind to yourself, and talk to people – when they ask, 'How are you?', tell them.

I am scared still, but that is not all I am, even though for a long time, it was pretty much all I knew and all I was.

CHAPTER 31

IN THE END...

I am passionate about the need to educate people about mental health and wellbeing and to break the stigma that stops people talking about it. It is a campaign that is gaining momentum but still has some way to go. I mentioned that during Mental Health Awareness Week in 2016 City AM, the Lord Mayor of London, Mind, The City Mental Health Alliance, Mental Health First Aid for England, Barclays Bank and others came together to promote This is Me in the City, an initiative to get people talking about the subject. I was asked to provide a profile, some of which I repeat below because it sums up so much of how I feel about the issue and why I am committed to it. It feels a good place to end.

My name is Richard Martin. I am 45 and a father of three. I am an employment lawyer by training. I enjoy all sorts of exercise and outdoor activity, DIY, cooking and reading. In 2011 I was hospitalised with anxiety and depression.

As a result of my work, I share my story freely. It took a bit of courage in the early days because I did not know how people would react, but the reaction has been hugely positive. People want to know. They sometimes think I am brave. I don't. It is much easier to be yourself than to try to pretend you are something else. When you are really ill, it can feel like ill is all you really are – it transcends everything. If you are unable to talk about it with people, friends and family especially, then you are shutting yourself off from people almost entirely. But human connection is vital to our wellbeing, whether we are ill or well. So, it is massively important to talk.

It's a truism that there remains a huge amount of stigma around mental ill health. Stigma comes from a lack of understanding, a lack of knowledge and insight. So, if we inform people we can start to break the stigma. And if we can get people who have suffered problems to talk about it then we break the taboo around the subject, we give people permission to talk about it, to normalise it in the way we have done with all sorts of other conditions. The This is Me campaign is all about that – normal people telling normal stories which happen to include the fact they suffer, or have suffered, from mental health problems. By showing others that they are just ordinary people like everyone else, and that their illness is fine to talk about, we remove the fear, the stigma, the taboo.

Since I was first ill I have read and studied a lot about how we think and feel and what makes people ill. Why do some people get ill and others not? There are a whole range of factors but what I have learnt more than anything else is that it is not events that cause us distress and problems but the way we react to them. And that is something we can try to understand and do something about. If I can understand the way my thinking works then I can challenge the less helpful elements and have a more balanced, a less stressful, reaction to events. And that will help me stay well. And this is something everyone can do, if only they knew about it, if only they had the information and the opportunity to think and talk about it.

I was delivering some awareness training recently to a group of senior in-house counsel. At the end of the session the only question was 'Why didn't we learn all this before?' And that's what I felt when I got ill. I did not see any of it coming. I was driving back from a holiday in France with my family and, apparently out of the blue, I had a huge panic attack. One day I am a successful lawyer, advising multinational clients and leading a team, the next I cannot leave the house, and am terrified of most things that happen in the house.

Over the weeks that followed my condition got worse until I ended up spending a month at the Priory. I was a complete wreck. Emotionally, and almost physically, I crawled into the Priory, desperate to escape from the world outside that terrified me.

Since then I have realised there were warning signs, it didn't come out of the blue, and that had I and those around me known more, then it might not have happened, or at least might not have got so bad.

It is five years on from my breakdown. I still suffer with anxiety and a bit of depression. I have quite a lot of flexibility over where and when I work which helps me to manage it. I also talk about it with my colleagues – when people ask me how I am, I think about the question and answer truthfully, rather than the normal "Fine". I have also learnt to be aware of, and to take heed of, my feelings – to recognise when I am feeling anxious and to think about why that is and what I can do about it. That's all about awareness.

I know how awful it is to suffer. I know what it is like to think that I cannot cope with being alive. I also know something of how awful it was for those around me to see me in that state. If just one person avoids that place because of this campaign, then it will have been worth it. If we get people talking about mental health, we can start educating people about how to look after themselves and each other, to keep well and to be alive to the warning signs and risk factors. We do it in every other aspect of our overall health, so why not our mental health?

Employers should get on board because they have the opportunity to make a difference, to create the environment in which this can happen. It is about creating a safe place and way to work, as well as looking after your primary assets, your people, promoting higher performance and productivity, and being kind. Why wouldn't you?

And, finally, something from my very early childhood, and a message to those that are suffering with mental health problems, or those who are caring for them.

Here we come, hand in hand,
Christopher Robin and I,
To lay this book in your lap.
Say you're surprised.
Say you like it.
Say it's just what you wanted.
Because it's yours,
Because we love you.

[AA Milne – To Her]

In the immortal words of Aretha Franklin, "I ain't no psychiatrist, I ain't no doctor with degree", but learning a little more about mental health and illness has been a key part of my recovery, and is now a vital part of my work, of course. If you are interested in reading more about that, I have created a website, www.richardmartinauthor.com, which contains much of that material and which, I hope, can be a living space and where I would be delighted to hear from any readers!

**If you found this book interesting ...
why not read these next?**

Teacup In A Storm

Finding My Psychiatrist

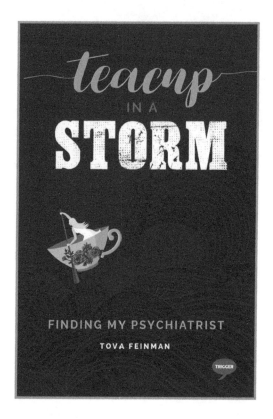

Wracked with trauma from childhood abuse, Tova sought
therapy to soothe her mind. However, it is not as easy as simply
finding a person to talk to ...

Stress in the City

Playing My Way Out of Depression

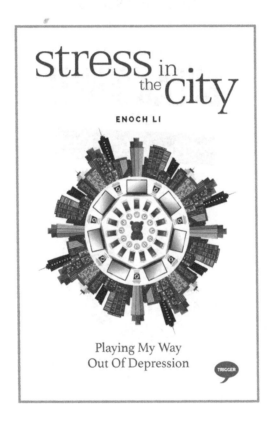

Stress in the City is a fascinating, information-packed self-help memoir, tackling the subjects of corporate pressure, depression and the benefits of playfulness within the recovery process.

Breakdown and Repair

A Businessman's Tale of Stress and Success

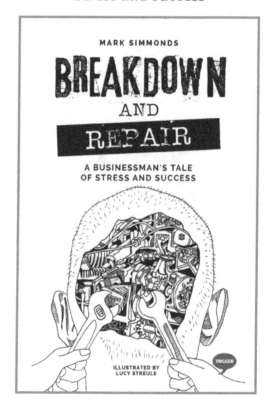

Succumbing to pressures from work, Mark pieces himself back together after attempting to take his own life. But he soon finds that it's not quite as easy as he might think, especially when his daughter takes a turn for the worst herself.

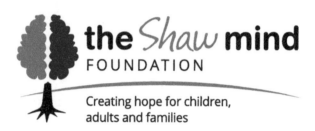

the *Shaw* mind
FOUNDATION

Creating hope for children,
adults and families

Sign up to our charity, The Shaw Mind Foundation
www.shawmindfoundation.org
and keep in touch with us; we would love to hear
from you.

*We aim to bring to an end the suffering and despair caused
by mental health issues. Our goal is to make help and support
available for every single person in society, from all walks of
life. We will never stop offering hope. These are our promises.*

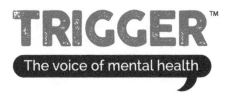

www.triggerpublishing.com

Trigger is a publishing house devoted to opening conversations about mental health. We tell the stories of people who have suffered from mental illnesses and recovered, so that others may learn from them.

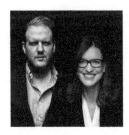

Adam Shaw is a worldwide mental health advocate and philanthropist. Now in recovery from mental health issues, he is committed to helping others suffering from debilitating mental health issues through the global charity he co-founded, The Shaw Mind Foundation. www.shawmindfoundation.org

Lauren Callaghan (CPsychol, PGDipClinPsych, PgCert, MA (hons), LLB (hons), BA), born and educated in New Zealand, is an innovative industry-leading psychologist based in London, United Kingdom. Lauren has worked with children and young people, and their families, in a number of clinical settings providing evidence based treatments for a range of illnesses, including anxiety and obsessional problems. She was a psychologist at the specialist national treatment centres for severe obsessional problems in the UK and is renowned as an expert in the field of mental health, recognised for diagnosing and successfully treating OCD and anxiety related illnesses in particular. In addition to appearing as a treating clinician in the critically acclaimed and BAFTA award-winning documentary *Bedlam*, Lauren is a frequent guest speaker on mental health conditions in the media and at academic conferences. Lauren also acts as a guest lecturer and honorary researcher at the Institute of Psychiatry Kings College, UCL.

Please visit the link below:

www.triggerpublishing.com

Join us and follow us...

@triggerpub

Search for us on Facebook